Resolute

MY QUEST FOR A NEW HEART

Resolute

LANCE J. CUNHA

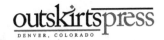
outskirtspress
DENVER, COLORADO

*Depicted on the cover is the author
four days after his heart transplant.*

Dedication

This book is dedicated principally to my wife, Mary. We fell in love as Freshmen at Ithaca College and, recently, celebrated 46 years of marriage. Despite being in <u>constant</u> pain from numerous/serious medical issues, Mary still **lived** this journey with me. As I waited for a heart for 2 ½ months in Emory University Hospital's Cardiac Care Unit (CCU), she spent virtually every day and night at my side. For this, and so much more, I'm eternally grateful.

This work is also dedicated to my daughters, Jennifer and Heather, their husbands, Heith and Christopher, and my dear grandchildren — Micah, Olivia, Alexander, Emory and William. Their visits, calls and thoughtfulness made me joyful and optimistic. Each of you in your own way encouraged me to think that I was never too old or too sick to achieve another goal or dream.

My CCU nurses and heart doctors must also be recognized. Their competence, consideration and caring made me believe that I could climb this mountain and make it to "the other side".

Finally, I must include my heart donor. He was a young man of 20 who, remarkably, had the maturity to give me the gift of life. Rest assured, I will invest wisely and lovingly in your – now my – strong and miraculous heart.

I love you all!

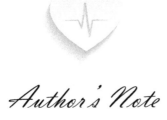

Author's Note

This memoir complements the *exceptionally beautiful* gift which my daughters, Jennifer and Heather, gave me for my 70th birthday. Their private and unpublished book, <u>Pass It On: Journey To A New Heart,</u> captures lovingly and poignantly six of the most critical months in my life. Displayed through their extraordinary photos, and exhibited through some elegant poems, messages and verses, are the significant roles my family played in keeping me alive. *Thank you, Jennifer and Heather.* <u>Pass It On...</u> will always be very special to our family and me.

Table of Contents

Prologue

On January 1, 2014, a young man and I "met" through a heart transplant. He was raised in a small town in Georgia; I in New York City. He had just died at age 20; I was rapidly approaching 69. This book covers how/where our lives intersected and the events leading up to that day. It's a story about utter sadness and glorious triumph; it's a memoir about my long/hard quest for a new heart; and it's a narrative of a man's resoluteness in seeking an impossible dream.

A principal factor driving my decision to write this book is to alert humanity to the life-saving importance of organ donations. My sincerest wish is that <u>Resolute...</u> will inspire many more people to become organ donors.

Another reason I'm making this effort is to help patients understand and anticipate better the difficult journeys of waiting for, hopefully receiving and then recovering from a heart transplant. I'm hopeful that <u>Resolute...</u> will help patients and their families find encouragement in my story and, by so doing, persevere.

A final reason I'm writing this book is to keep my promise to God, my immediate family and dearest friends. I believe that **all** encouraged me to commit pen to paper by describing these miraculous events in my life. As I considered writing <u>Resolute...</u>, I struggled for months with the agonizing emotional challenges I knew I would encounter if/as I revisited this remarkable voyage. Nevertheless, 18 months after my heart transplant, I arrived at the conclusion that this story <u>must</u> be told.

Lance J. Cunha
Johns Creek, GA
January 2016

Note to Readers

Throughout <u>Resolute...</u>, I have used interchangeably the words doctor, doc. and docs. No disrespect was ever intended. Along this journey, I became very comfortable with the Medical Doctors who were – and still are – caring for me. Given our close relationships, I called some doc. and, a few, even by their familiar names. Similarly in this book, whenever I've referred to my pharmaceutical needs, I've used reciprocally the words medications, meds. and prescriptions. Whichever word came to mind first was utilized at the moment I was writing.

CHAPTER I:
The Initial Diagnosis

In 1970, with a freshly-minted Master's Degree from the University of Notre Dame, I began my career on Wall Street. I was 25 years old and felt invincible. I had been married for less than a year to my college sweetheart and, for the first time in my life, had some money in my pocket. Most importantly, I was an international banker and, finally, would begin to live my dreams of world travel and helping less developed countries.

Over the next 34 years, as a banker and consultant, I worked in over 50 countries. At times, some of those countries were among the poorest on earth. In addition to working in the world's capital markets, I also traveled to places such as the jungles of South America and Southeast Asia. The latter exposed me to some serious health risks. Save the severe health "consequences" later in my life, I have never had any regrets as to my life's work and extensive travels. The "consequences", first appearing in 2004, were the early stages of *heart failure*.

In early October 2004, while living in New Canaan, Connecticut, I saw my local Primary Care Provider (PCP). I hadn't felt well for several months and was always out-of-breath, fatigued and bloated. Frequently, it seemed, I also suffered from "colds" and related respiratory problems. After being examined by my PCP, he urged me to see a local/prominent cardiologist. The latter, noting my risks professionally (in particular my work in less developed countries), as well as my family's background of heart disease, had me evaluated thoroughly by his team at Connecticut's Norwalk Hospital. Naturally, to determine clearly the condition of my heart, my doctors included extensive blood work, stress testing and an echocardiogram and angiogram.

Within a week of my cardiological evaluations, my cardiologist sent me a detailed letter. In that letter he described my condition as a "hypertrophic cardiomyopathy" (essentially, an enlarged heart). He recommended stress reduction, less travel, decreasing my sodium intake and, if possible, a move to a warmer climate. The latter to mitigate the risks of cold weather and their deleterious effects on my breathing and enlarged/overworked heart. At 59 years old, I was told that, in order to save my life, my work habits would have to change significantly.

Since my older daughter was already settled in the Atlanta area, Mary and I decided that I would "semi-retire" and, despite our solid "Yankee" roots, we would move south.

Over the next four years from my Georgia home I consulted for a few major banks. Simultaneously, Mary and I focused diligently on selling our New Canaan, Connecticut home and enjoying our two young grandchildren, Micah and Olivia (born in 2003 and 2004, respectively). Through a friend, I had established a relationship with a local cardiologist at Atlanta's Piedmont Hospital. Although ostensibly concerned about my deteriorating heart failure symptoms, my Piedmont doctor insisted on treating them solely with medications. From time-to-time, I questioned his complacency and lack of proactivity regarding my care. However, I stayed the course until, in the late fall of 2007, I became very sick. My symptoms included chest congestion/discomfort and difficulty breathing. After three visits to my PCP, I insisted on a chest x-ray. The latter, taken on January 9, 2008, indicated that I was extremely ill and probably in danger of death from congestive heart failure.

My PCP advised me to be seen by a different cardiologist as soon as possible.

From the time Mary and I moved to Georgia, I deeply regret not seeking advice immediately from Dr. Andrew Smith and his heart failure colleagues at Emory University Hospital (EUH). In-time, however, Providence would lead me to EUH.

CHAPTER II:

"My Heart Is Shot"

*"Inside every older person is a younger person
wondering what the hell happened"*

—Author unknown

My grandson, Alexander, was born in New York City on January 13, 2008. Two days after Alexander's birth, Mary and I were in "The Big Apple". While there, I received an urgent phone call from my Atlanta PCP who urged me to return home immediately. At his discretion, that PCP had asked a cardiologist (but not my Piedmont doc.!) to review my x-rays and his recent medical notes. The new cardiologist indicated to my PCP that I was in extreme duress and, based on the x-rays, I was in grave danger of possibly dying soon from a heart attack.

That message utterly shocked Mary and me. Holding my new grandson (and thinking about my other two grandchildren), I felt very upset and confused. Within two days, Mary and I cautiously returned to Atlanta. When we arrived, I was admitted promptly to St. Joseph's Hospital. The new cardiologist had arranged for me to have multiple tests to determine the exact condition of my heart and what course of action should be taken. The results of the testing were sobering; to save my life, the doctor advised my wife that I "must have surgery <u>immediately</u> for implantation of a pacemaker and defibrillator". He added: "your husband's been sedated and, given his critical condition, he cannot leave the hospital". He then urged Mary to call our family and let them know of my very serious condition.

With two nurses observing me constantly, and Mary and Jennifer at my bedside, the new cardiologist then explained to me as well that *my heart is shot.* My Ejection Fraction (EF)* was hovering around 20, and my heart was in imminent risk of failing. Yet, much to my family's amazement (but, for me, quite typical!), I insisted on a "second opinion" before allowing surgery. However, my daughter and wife took charge and, without hesitation, overruled

---

*   Ejection Fraction (EF) is the fraction of outbound blood pumped from the heart with each heartbeat.

me and told the doctor to move forward. Thankfully, on that day, my pacemaker and defibrillator were "installed". Undoubtedly, that urgent procedure saved my life! My operation was followed immediately by new/stronger medications which, juxtaposing my pacemaker and de-fibrillator, would help regulate and protect my severely damaged heart.

The e-mail which follows summarizes quite well "My Condition" up to and at that time. It was sent to my immediate family on February 7, 2008 after I recovered from the life-changing events of the previous month.

> I discovered recently that, for all or most of my life, I've had what's known as an 'athlete's heart'. The official term is hypertrophic cardiomyopathy. Essentially, my heart was not as elastic as it should be. Therefore, if attacked or infected, my heart was incapable of responding as well as most. Adding to the problem, was my heart's thickness. To try to compensate for its lack of elasticity, my heart has gradually become much thicker. Any muscle which is taxed will grow until, of course, it is injured or, in my case, "fails".

Now let's focus on the present. A virus has attacked my heart and caused significant damage. Perhaps, absent the cardiomyopathy, my heart might have been able to resist the virus. However, for whatever reason, that virus has caused grave and irreparable cardiac damage. The lower chambers (especially the left ventricle) were compromised the most and, given their ongoing disfunctionality, my ejection fraction (EF) has fallen dangerously low. Where ordinarily the EF should be in the 60-65 range, with me it has fallen to 20. With an EF of 20, the physicians were amazed that I could even walk!

Today, I'm living with *Heart Failure.* In a nutshell that means that my heart has lost its ability to pump properly. The pacemaker and defibrillator in my chest are designed to help keep me alive.

Now why am I telling you all of this? Principally because I want to be open with you with respect to why, from time-to-time, I may be less energetic. My EF, meds., exercise and stress may affect my moods, concentration and daily functionality. Hopefully, in time (probably/eventually with a heart transplant), I'll be able to reacquire some of what I used to be able to do.

Hence, in earnest, began my nearly 6 year journey to live!

CHAPTER III:

Searching For Hope

*"You may not control events that happen to you,
but you can decide not to be reduced by them"*

—*Maya Angelou*

B eginning in 2008, Mary and I began to consider solutions for my deteriorating health. For most of 2008, my body had to adjust to my new meds. and slower pace of life. Then, unfortunately, in October Mary had a near death experience following a disastrous thyroidectomy. The latter, performed by a cavalier Atlanta surgeon, required two evacuations to stop the bleeding. The collateral damages since then have been <u>catastrophic</u> to Mary's health. Yet, as Mary recovered gradually, our priorities in 2009 became my heart and, as such, we were desperate for advice.

Through a contact in New Canaan we were introduced to a very prominent heart failure doctor at The Cleveland Clinic. The latter is the #1 cardiac hospital in the U.S. Therefore, in the spring of 2010, after several months of discussions, completing and forwarding detailed medical information, etc., Mary and I traveled to Cleveland to be examined by that notable cardiologist and his team.

At The Cleveland Clinic, three days were devoted to the most thorough examinations of my life. Nothing was overlooked; tests and more tests were completed. Quite graciously, the heart failure doctors stayed with me throughout the process.

After those three challenging days, it was confirmed that I was in Stage 3 heart failure. The numbers were not encouraging and, diplomatically, the doctors told Mary and me that I was "in a downward spiral". Four suggestions were made. Namely, to: (i) see the heart failure/transplant team at Emory University Hospital (EUH); (ii) look into the University of Miami's work in stem cells; (iii) adopt more aggressive diuretic therapy; and (iv) reduce my stress levels. We embraced all 4 suggestions simultaneously.

Within weeks of my trip to The Cleveland Clinic, I contacted EUH's heart failure team. Thankfully, I was admitted promptly to EUH's heart failure practice.

That summer, after reviewing all of my records from Piedmont Hospital (where I had also been treated) and, of course, The Cleveland Clinic, my Emory docs. decided "to be proactive" in my care. I welcomed that approach wholeheartedly and, thus, began the arduous task of EUH determining if, at age 65, I might be eligible for a heart transplant.

By the summer of 2011, Mary and I had already made three trips to the University of Miami to explore stem cells to treat my rapidly weakening heart. Each time, I was evaluated and tested in every conceivable way. Initially, there was optimism that I would qualify for the stem cell research trials. The results had been dramatic with others (50% increases or more in their EFs) – and, save my heart, I was in pretty good shape. Mary and I rejoiced at this news and began to sense that stem cells might be the solution. When we informed my Emory docs., they, too, felt that this simultaneous path to survival was "worth exploring".

Yet, early in the New Year, heartbreaking news arrived. On January 19, 2012, I was informed that I would not be eligible for stem cell trials. The National Institutes of Health (NIH) which were funding the stem cell study/ research project required an ejection fraction higher than mine. I sensed that the University of Miami felt that my extremely low EF might be more difficult to increase and, thus, have a deleterious effect on the trials' overall statistics/results. This was a terrible shock to Mary and me; no one had ever mentioned that specific measure/criteria to us. We felt misled by/very angry with Miami's docs. More importantly, as days passed, we became more apprehensive than ever before as to our chances for a life-saving solution in-time to save my life.

2012 passed quickly. The frequency and exigency of doctors' appointments at EUH intensified. I knew things were getting worse as, on three occasions, I had collapsed and been hospitalized for dangerously low blood pressure and other related/serious complications. In one of those instances, my defibrillator had actually fired and, by so doing, probably saved my life!

Still that fall, despite me feeling poorly, Mary and I made the voyage by plane and car to Ithaca, NY. Ithaca College had chosen to honor me with its highest alumni award. Namely, for "Lifetime Achievement". Heather's family joined us in Ithaca and made it an even more memorable event.

During 2012, some of our close friends in New Canaan, CT had either died or become very sick. Therefore, at the last minute, we decided to spend New Year's Eve with some of our most intimate friends. On December 30 and 31st, we drove 960 miles straight through from Georgia to Connecticut. We arrived at some dear friends' home on the afternoon of December 31st . There we napped, showered and dressed in black tie for New Year's Eve. As a complete surprise to our other friends, we arrived at the Country Club of New Canaan in-time to dine and celebrate heartily the 2012 New Year. At midnight, exhausted from the drive, I remember whispering to Mary that I was savoring the evening. At that moment, I also recall feeling that this could be the last time I would spend a New Year celebration with my wife and these wonderful people. Little did I know that, one year later, I'd be about to receive a miracle!

CHAPTER IV:
Tempting Providence

"The policy of being too cautious is the greatest risk of all"

—*Jawaharlal Nehru*

For almost 44 years I had promised Mary that, some-day, I would dance the waltz with her in Vienna, Austria. Although we had traveled to count-less countries, for several reasons we had never been to Austria. Therefore, despite my weakened condition and ignoring doctors' advice, I decided to book us on a July 2013 Danube River Cruise. However, before leaving, my doctor insisted on two important "details".

First, that my pacemaker and defibrillator be upgraded. That required surgery and, in light of my extremely low EF, any surgery was very risky. Moreover, when upgraded, electrical complications with my delicate heart leads could cause arrhythmias and even possible death.

Second, I was required to complete the eligibility process to be added to the heart transplant list. By then, save a kidney biopsy, I had met (and passed) all of the complicated and tedious eligibility requirements (physical, emotional, psychological, etc.). Therefore, in late June, I had a kidney biopsy to ensure that my kidneys were functioning at 92% or higher.

My kidney biopsy involved two large needles being inserted into my back one at a time. The needles needed to be guided carefully around my ribs and into my kidneys. Save Lidocain at the entry site, no other medication was administered. The needle was quite intimidating and the test itself quite painful, especially when the docs. hit a rib!

Nevertheless, after flying to Budapest (via London), our 10 day river cruise was fabulous! From Budapest, Hungary to Prague, Czech Republic (and including glorious stops in Austria and Germany), the sites, history, charm and beauty of the Danube and the cities, towns and villages near same were utterly magnificent. And yes, indeed, I danced the waltz with my bride in Vienna! Adding to my joy was an e-mail I received confirming that I had passed the kidney tests and was "eligible" for the Heart Transplant List.

In August 2013, Mary and I made an emergency trip to New York City for a week to help our younger daughter, Heather, her husband, Christopher, and their sons, Alexander and William. Heather was recovering from a cancer-caused thyroidectomy and subsequent harsh reactions to radiation treatment and new medications. Albeit at home, Heather was quite sick and very weak. At the time, Alexander was 5 and William was just learning to walk. Very kindly, our older daughter, Jennifer, had preceded us to N.Y. for a week to care for/help Heather. However, Jennifer had to return to Roswell, GA to prepare her children for the new school year. Christopher had a demanding job on Wall Street and could not take any more time off from his job. Therefore, with only a moment's notice, we packed a couple of bags and drove to N.Y. Albeit exhausting given our ages and poor health, if necessary we would do it again in a *heartbeat* for either of our daughters. We call that life-long parental "bench strength".

In October 2013, fearing the worst, I told Mary that I wanted to visit Los Cabos, Mexico. Mary and I had been to Mexico several times, but never to Los Cabos. The real truth was that I knew I was very sick and wanted quiet time alone with Mary to reflect on our lives and, hopefully, allow her to concentrate on our estate planning, asset management, and other (mostly financial) advice. Although more than ever before, my doctors weighed in negatively, I knew that if I stayed home Mary would be distracted and the "just-in-case" notes which I prepared largely ignored. However, as we landed in Cabo San Lucas, I wondered if this would be my last trip. Was I destined to die in Mexico?

I booked us for a week at the beautiful Los Cabos Hilton Resort. The week was fabulous and relaxing! Every day, the sun, sand and sea made us feel as if we were on our honeymoon. Although I was too weak to walk to the ocean or even on the beach, I did spend hours each day strolling in the pool. Perhaps, in part, because I was an American who had worked hard to learn Spanish well, the staff in many ways went out of their way to treat Mary and me very kindly and graciously.

On October 23, 2013, one day after returning from Los Cabos and in grave condition, I was admitted to EUH's CCU. Coincidentally, a month earlier, my daughters had raised a large flag in the front yard of my home. On that flag were inscribed the words: "Don't Give Up The Ship". That slogan, of course taken from Commodore Perry's battle flag in the War of 1812, encouraged me to have courage and, now in the CCU, fight for my life. It also reminded me of an impressionable quote from my Roman History and Altar Boy/Latin studies: "Qui Transluit Sustinet" ("He who brought us here will care for us").

CHAPTER V:
Some Reality Checks

A s an economist by education, training and experience, I immediately began to research heart transplant statistics, related probabilities and prognoses. What I discovered was quite unsettling! I learned, for instance, that there are approximately 123,000 people in the U.S. waiting urgently for organ transplantation. Every year most, without an imminent match, would probably not survive. Each year, of those waiting, most do not receive their miracles. Principal reason: a paucity of organ donors. Of those waiting for a heart transplant, the percentages of these marvels relative to those waiting are even lower. Why? It seems that the heart is often the most difficult for a family to donate. Culturally and spiritually, this is partially understandable. The heart is revered and, of course, holidays such as Valentine's Day, Mother's Day, engagements, weddings, births, etc. awaken unique heart-related sentiments. Additionally, throughout history, the heart and soul have often been linked closely in various religious and cultural rituals. Therefore, although other organs may be donated, sometimes there are emotional strings tied to the heart which discourage its harvesting and transplantation.

Also complicating heart transplantation is that the time period for a heart transplant is only about 4 hours. That means that no more than 4 hours should elapse between harvesting and transplanting a heart. That logistical requirement makes heart transplantation even more difficult. Virtually from the time a potential donor is declared brain dead, his/her body is kept "alive" artificially. An experienced harvest team is sent immediately from a recipient's hospital to the donor's hospital. Even before the harvest team arrives, the local doctors begin (very respectfully) to withdraw blood, tissue samples, etc. to begin to determine the best match among those on the waiting list. All involved, pray that the donor's heart will be a match for someone.

From the time the harvest team arrives at the donor's bedside, it will be in constant contact with its surgical colleagues at the recipient's hospital. Everything is examined, reviewed and verified multiple times to ensure maximum compatibility between the donor and potential recipient. Only when it's a "go", is the likelihood of a heart transplant confirmed to a desperately anxious patient/recipient and his/ her family.

Noteworthy is the sensitivity with which the donor's family is counseled through this entire/very difficult ordeal. Well-trained professionals from the Donate Life organizations (in my case, Donate Life Georgia) are with the deceased family <u>constantly</u>. That team, as well as appropriate clerical personnel, do God's work on the scene by helping a family cope with the unimaginable (often sudden) loss of a loved one. Ordinarily the family will respect their loved one's wishes and, with great anguish, allow the harvest team to proceed.

Given the tight schedule between harvesting and transplantation, all potential donor recipients are situated in one of 11 regions in the U.S. I was in the southeastern region (Region #3). That meant that, despite my critical/top priority 1A status*, my heart donor would have to come from one of a handful of states in the southeast or Puerto Rico. There would be no exceptions to these UNOS (United Network for Organ Sharing) geographic protocols. Since

---

*   1A designates the most critical need for a heart transplant.

in every region (save Alaska and Hawaii) demand for organs far exceeded availability, I inquired specifically about
the numbers at EUH. Disappointingly, I discovered that in
2012 fewer than 50 heart transplants had been performed.
Even more discouraging, however, I learned that, as of
October 23, 2013 (the date of my admission to the CCU),
only approximately half that number had so far been ac-
complished in 2013.

Another significant challenge for those waiting for a
heart transplant is the disproportionate number of possible
recipients versus potential donors. At the same time over
5.7 million Americans are living with heart failure and
670,000 new cases are diagnosed each year. Quite tragi-
cally, the gap between those waiting for a heart and the
pool of donors widens each year.

Age, too, is an important factor in heart transplantation. Eligibility for anyone over 60, will find it much more
difficult to qualify. Everything is tested to ensure that any
potential recipient meets strict eligibility requirements.
As one ages, "things" deteriorate and weaken. Hence, it's
even more difficult for those over 60 "to make the cut". In
all fairness, however, I agree with UNOS' requirements.
An older man or woman must be: (a) healthy enough (save
his/her heart, of course) to survive a heart transplant; and

(b) expected to have a chance of living at least long enough to have justified giving him/her a heart instead of to someone younger.

After trying to absorb all this information, Mary and I had great trepidation as to my real chances of ever receiving the miracle of a new heart. Based on the statistics and probabilities, the prognoses were not good. The odds were definitely against me. Nevertheless, I reasoned, the alternative was unacceptable! After all, I loved my family too much and wanted to witness my 5 exceptional grandchildren grow and prosper. Therefore, to live, I knew that I would have to fight valiantly!

CHAPTER VI:

CCU-409

*"Never give up, for that is the time
and place that the tide will turn"*

—Harriet Beecher Stowe

On October 23, 2013, quite early in the morning, Mary and I arrived at EUH's Catheter Lab. I had been scheduled for several tests – including an angiogram, echocardiogram, etc. As my doctor proceeded, he suddenly became <u>very</u> concerned. Without any warning, he ordered me transferred to the CCU "stat". My heart was about to fail!

As three technicians raced me on a stretcher from the Cath. Lab to the CCU, they were literally flying through the halls. One technician's only job was to make sure that

I didn't fall off the stretcher. Mary was told that I was in extreme danger and that she should merely follow the stretcher. But Mary couldn't keep up and, shouting to the technicians, demanded to know where they were taking me. The answer – the hospital's CCU/4G.

The CCU is a dedicated intensive care unit for only critically ill heart patients. Limited to a dozen or so patients at any one time, several were waiting for heart transplants. Within minutes of my arrival in CCU-409, I was stripped of my clothing, given a hospital gown and hooked-up intravenously to several drugs. The admitting nurses (one quite serious, the other with a calming/engaging smile) were quite efficient and seemed to be following a rigid protocol. Although confused, alarm only emerged when I saw Mary and my principal cardiac doctor's grim faces.

I met my principal cardiac doctor at EUH soon after my Cleveland Clinic visit. I liked him immediately. He was the doctor who, at our first meeting, told me that he wanted to be "proactive" in my care. My response at that time: you're hired! As we became acquainted, I asked him to keep me alive until his young daughters' weddings. I promised that if we built this "living annuity" together, I would give each daughter a very nice gift at her wedding. That cardiac doctor had guided me through the eligibility process and teed me up for a heart transplant. I saw kindness in his eyes and, despite his carefully starched appearance and sterling credentials, he had a quick sense of humor. Notwithstanding his claims to be a "worker bee", I enjoyed telling him that he was on his way to becoming a heart failure "luminary". However, on that October day, I saw in him a man about to tell his patient that things looked gloomy and grim.

My doctor advised me that I was "gravely ill". He added that, if I left the hospital, my chances of survival would be very low. At any moment, my heart was in danger of completely stopping. However, since I had met all the eligibility requirements for a heart transplant, if I stayed in the hospital's CCU waiting for a heart I would be classified as 1A. That meant that I would be among those near the top of the regional (southeastern) transplant list. Until a heart became available, I would be kept alive on a drug called Milrinone and several other powerful drugs. When I asked if there was a "Plan B", I was told that I could go home, get/stay hooked-up intravenously by Mary, and hope that there would not be any "emergent" situations. When I asked my doctor what he meant by "emergent situations", he mentioned possible infections, ambulances, Emergency Rooms and, naturally, the greater threat of congestive heart failure and death. Additionally, if I chose

Plan B, I would be categorized 1B rather than 1A. The difference in status was the result of non-medically trained care at home versus full-time (24/7) preparation and readiness by my CCU doctors and nurses. Much to Mary and my doctor's enormous surprise, I asked for a few minutes to think about my options.

My immediate concerns related to utter confinement for an undefined period of time. I also needed to know that my family could visit regularly. Much to my doctor's amazement, I asked for "statistics" as to how long this "incarceration" might last. His answers were as follows: (i) "yes" — that unless they were sick my family would have full visitation privileges; and (ii) although "timing was up to God", given my A+ blood type (second most common), the statistics were in my favor for a shorter wait. I also inquired about the drugs, side effects and their administration. A nurse gave me a list of the drugs (already ordered), mentioned possible collateral problems and told me that a Swan Ganz Pulmonary Artery Catheter ("Swan") holding multiple ports would be inserted in my neck. The nurse added, quite emphatically (as Mary pressured me to stay), that the collateral problems, discomfort (really a metaphor for pain!), Swan, etc. should be considered a "better alternative to dying". Agreeing, I decided to go ahead with the program and surrender to whatever would follow. Hence began a dark/ unspecific journey – one which would lead to one of three outcomes: (i) a miracle (i.e., a new heart); (ii) a Left Ventricular Assist Device (LVAD) to try to "bridge" my wait for a new heart; or (iii) death. Mary and I hugged, shed a few tears and, with this sobering "news", called our daughters, my brother and Mary's sister and brother.

CCU-409 was a small, compact room. A toilet existed, but it was about 8 feet away from my bed. The toilet was only reachable with help from a technician or nurse. It often took a nurse or technician at least 8 minutes from the time of my "call" to rearrange all my plugs, tubes and cords to allow me to cross the room and make it to the "throne". Of course, my "comfort station" was available for bowel movements only; everything else was collected pertinaciously to measure my fluid levels. My diet was regimented and liquids of any kind (including those from fruit, soup, etc.) were monitored carefully. The daily menu was virtually the same – boring and unseasoned. Dinner "specials" were announced each morning – but, they too, were monotonous. Most of the time I ordered very plain comfort foods; my appetite was nonexistent.

The tightness in CCU-409 was exacerbated by the devices, equipment, tubes, Ivs, etc. hooked-up to my body.

They were everywhere! I was prohibited from getting out of bed unless I had help. Early on that agitated me; however, as time passed and I became weaker, I understood those important "risk management" protocols.

CCU-409 had no windows. My only hope at sunlight was a small corridor behind the guests' access door at the rear of my room. Given the difficulty to move all my equipment, I sat out there only once. Gradually, I grew pale from the lack of sun and poor circulation. Additionally, there was no incentive to venture out. Privacy disallowed any patient-to-patient contact. Nevertheless, three of us waiting for a heart transplant ignored those instructions and, occasionally, called each other's room by phone just to chat. With humor and song, I tried to stimulate laughter, small talk about goals and, in general, positive conversation. For most waiting for a heart transplant, depression was a <u>huge</u> problem!

One of the stories I shared with a few of my "neighbors" was an e-mail I received when I first arrived in CCU-409. It was from a life insurance broker. It indicated that I "was underinsured and needed more life insurance". I had no idea how this broker got my name or why she felt that I needed more protection. Nevertheless, after I called my doctors and nurses into my room for a chuckle, I decided to play along. I told the broker that "I agreed" and, yes, indeed, I could use another million or two in life insurance. But first, I thought I should be candid and tell her where I was and why I was there. Hilariously, a few days later, the broker's response was to offer me an accidental death policy! Perhaps she was thinking that I might fall out of bed or off a stretcher.

Another "story" related to the "Red Phone". This wonderful myth began when I was a young Altar Boy. One day, when I was very upset (not uncommon since I had a tormenting, abusive and ignorant mother), a priest told me that in difficult times I must be alert for God's miraculous Red Phone. The latter, the priest added, would be "there" for me if I listened for it carefully. Throughout my personal and professional lives, in some very challenging situations, I "heard" the Red Phone ring. It gave me strength and courage and helped me find the right path forward. In the CCU, I spoke of the Red Phone virtually every day. All the CCU nurses, some doctors and a few patients quickly learned what it meant. I encouraged some patients to allow their senses to be alert for the unique chimes of God's Red Phone. I conveyed the omnipresence of the Red Phone and its message of faith and hope. I asked the nurses regularly to make sure that when – not if – the Red phone rang, answer it promptly. I counseled them never to allow that call to go to voice mail. After all, the miraculous toll will signal that a heart for one of us was on its way!

As I mentioned earlier in this Chapter, depression was a chronic problem with most of the heart transplant patients. Despondency was increased dramatically and palpably when someone died. We all knew; the curtains would be drawn and the nurses' station would be very somber. In my CCU "class" I was the oldest. Nevertheless, a few died while I was waiting and another (one of those with whom I had chatted regularly by phone) committed suicide three weeks after my heart transplant. He was 52, had been waiting for almost 4 months and, according to his nurses, "just given up". (My other principal contact by phone, received a heart on Palm Sunday 2014. Thankfully he's doing quite well.) In that context, it would have been timely, thoughtful and, perhaps, life-saving if a psychologist visited each CCU patient regularly. Although Chaplains, etc. occasionally made the rounds, a bright and caring Ph.D. psychologist to counsel patients might have helped to alleviate for some patients their depression, loneliness, anxiety and/or hopelessness.

Along the same lines as the absence of a psychologist, I was astonished that neither of my two/probable transplant surgeons ever visited me. By visiting my room, and discussing openly the heart transplant process, a surgeon's visit would have been reassuring and informative for both my family and me. To no avail, my several requests were ignored (including an Emory Portal Message directly to the senior heart transplant surgeon).

Save the last week when I was transferred to a larger room on the 3rd floor (CCU-409 was on the 4th floor), CCU-409 would be my home until a matching heart arrived. That very thought, namely waiting for a man to die so that I could live, troubled me frequently. I wondered if the match would be good and what life might be like with another man's heart.* I considered the circumstances which would cause death (often sudden) to an organ donor and the pain that the family would endure. Yet, I still yearned for the trip to "the other side": the post-transplant ICU.

The Swan was one of the most difficult parts of my circumscription. It's a device inserted into my neck and coming to rest in my pulmonary artery. Typically, there are multiple ports attached to the Swan – each, through the Swan, feeding different meds. directly into my body. The Swan replaced the need for multiple Iv sites and, for both patients and nurses, facilitated the timing and delivery of

---

*   If success is defined as survival for several years, a heart transplant should be gender specific.

medications. At any time, I had as many as 8 ports affixed to my Swan. The Swan is a strict UNOS requirement while waiting for a heart transplant.

The insertion of the Swan was always very painful. It was worse when it was done by a "Fellow" rather than a seasoned cardiac doctor. The best to perform this procedure would have been one of my nurses. Indeed, two nurses in particular seemed much more experienced and qualified. Often, after insertion, those nursing angels would adjust my Swan into a more comfortable position. Moreover, every two-three days or so, these special nurses would remove the bandages in the areas adjacent to my Swan and, gently and tenderly, clean my neck. That process was sheer joy as my neck often itched badly from both the bandages and constant irritation.

But the protocols for Swan insertion were that it must be handled by an M.D. – irrespective of the doctor's experience. Since EUH is a teaching hospital, I had to submit to allowing young doctors (i.e., Fellows) to manhandle me for the sake of learning. Afterwards, however, I often enjoyed teasing those Fellows about their "indelicate hands".

The principal problem with the Swan was the risk of staph infection. If an infection was contracted, it would cause high fever and, possibly, death. It could also make me temporarily ineligible if a heart arrived. During my 70 day wait, I had to endure three horrible staph infections. Because of my weak heart, each required urgent antibiotic remedies. Each time with a staph infection the Swan was removed. I'd bleed some and, as always, simply surrender to the pain. Thankfully, the staph infections (including the tortuous side-effects) lasted for only about 4 days. However, in the meantime, the Swan needed to be replaced with something else. That's when I got to know of Picc Lines and a very special Catheter (Cath.) Technician.

A Picc Line is a device used instead of a Swan. It functions as a Swan – but, instead of a neck insertion, it's placed under your arm. Given the location (i.e., through soft tissue under the arm), Picc Line insertion is also quite painful. Since 1A heart transplant patients must at all times have either a Swan or a Picc Line, I bit the bullet each time either was "installed" and, during the ordeal, suffered in silence.

Sleeping with either a Swan or Picc Line was also very difficult. It was impossible to get comfortable. Often, instead of reclining fully, I would sleep in an upright position. I'd struggle to find a way to decrease my discomfort and avoid the device's irritating side-effects. Many nights, even sleep medication could not mitigate the annoyances caused by my Swan or Picc Line.

Whenever a Picc Line was needed, I insisted on a specialized Cath.Technician. Describing the man I preferred is difficult. He was quite muscular, in his late 30s, wore a bandana, rode a motorcycle and had an ear ring. My initial impression was that he seemed too tough for this job. However, I was wrong! Actually, that Cath. Technician was bright and, given his caring demeanor, well-suited for his job – and for me! Most importantly, he had "soft hands" and, as time went on, I considered him a true blessing. I cherish a photo taken of us, and I certainly hope to see him again someday.

From the first week, Mary was permitted to have a fold-up cot in my room. A Walmart purchase by my daughter, Jennifer, the cot allowed Mary to sleep somewhat comfortably at night. The alternative would have been an uncomfortable reclining chair. For those 70 tense days, Mary was with me virtually every day and night. Not a day went by that I didn't feel guilty about Mary's dedication. I worried constantly about her health and, often redundantly, reminded her of doctors' appointments, med. schedules, etc.

My daughter, Jennifer, and her family visited frequently; her husband, Heith, also stopped-by regularly on his lunch breaks. Very thoughtfully, Jennifer brought me permissible snacks (including my favorite candies) and, on two occasions, excellent sushi. Heather and her husband, Chris, sent me a case of low sodium soup* and, when Heather was in-town, she always got me Dunkin Donuts coffee and blueberry muffins. My cousin, Keith, his wife, Cathy, and their entire family also visited regularly and, characteristically, were always available to help and support my immediate family's emotional and logistical needs. I'll always be most grateful to them for their kindness and generosity.

Many friends also visited. However, their stays were usually truncated by my nurses. Impolitely sometimes, I fell asleep and Mary had to fill in the blanks. Special surprises were the unexpected visits of two "old" friends, Ira Kent and Richard Dubbs (aka "Dubbs"). I'd known Ira since our freshmen year at Ithaca College; Richard had been a colleague of mine in the 1980s at Manufacturers Hanover (today part of JPMorgan Chase). Ira flew up from Florida; Richard traveled south from N.Y. Ira and I reminisced about our life-long ping pong tournaments and, with a confident smile, I told him I'd be back! Since

---

*   Heather (at the time living in NYC) ordered this soup by phone from Trader Joe's, a local merchant in Marietta, GA. When my cousin, Keith (residing in Marietta), picked-up the case of soup to take to me, the store's manager – knowing from Heather the soup's purpose and destination – told Keith that there would be no charge!

I had enjoyed many years of college football with Richard (a University of Southern California graduate), he commissioned for me an official Notre Dame football jersey (including, on the back, my name and number 1). These are good and thoughtful men and, as close friends, they have always been very special to me.

When the grandchildren visited it was always an adventure. My granddaughter, Emory,* for instance (then 4), seeing her name everywhere, asked if she was famous. I told her, of course! Olivia, then 9, told me that "they couldn't take my heart because that's where all my love was". Alexander, then 5, played soccer in the hallway behind my room. Goals were constructed and sometimes, to my nurses' chagrin, Alexander would shout "GOAL". William, then 1, played in bed with me and, as he belly laughed, we threw ice chips into cups in each other's laps. With sheer joy, William also relished trying all the hand sanitizers he could find on the floor. Since Micah, then 10, had a school paper due on my family's heritage, it gave us an excellent opportunity (in-person and by e-mail) to work closely together. My grandkids brought me great joy and, through that inner contentment, a way to

---

*   My daughter, Jennifer, and her husband Heith, met and fell in love at Emory Law School. Hence their youngest child (also, possibly, a lawyer someday!) was named Emory.

allow my mind to relax.* In addition to learning something from them, I hope I demonstrated to them something important about their G-Dad's courage and character. Based on my **ten year-old** grandson/Micah's essay, I made an impression! (Exactly as written, Micah's essay is included as Appendix A.)

The most unique items in my room were the posters and pictures which embellished all of my walls. No other room resembled mine. Soon after my arrival in CCU-409, Jennifer had beautiful posters made with family photos and special events. Heather, too, contributed meaningfully to same. Of course, of special interest to me was my grandchildren's "artwork"! Some of that artwork was actually colored lovingly by my grandkids in the hallway behind my room. Every inch of my walls was covered in photos, notes, cards and drawings. The room's décor became a testimony to my family's love, closeness and support. Around the holidays (Halloween, Thanksgiving and Christmas), my room was also decorated very festively with new "artwork" and, as permitted, beautiful seasonal items. As Christmas approached, Mary and some friends added two small/beautiful Christmas trees and tasteful decorations to brighten my spirits.

---

* My daughter, Heather, a Ph.D. Psychologist, also helped me with some subtle, but very timely, messages and advice.

The days were long and the nights endless! Despite sleeping medication, I had great difficulty sleeping. I was haunted by uncertainty; the night's silence was deafening; and, at times, the demons minatory. I was unafraid of death, but agonized at the thought of missing my wife, children and grandchildren. Sometimes, I spent the entire night reliving my life and, with a few regrets, playing over and over some mistakes I had made. At those times, however, I would gain strength from Robert Frost: "The woods are lovely, dark and deep ...but I have promises to keep and miles to go before I sleep". But the pounding in my head always told me I was still alive. Each day, my early morning medications and some cheery nurses revived me and, with new determination, I pushed on.

Mary, too, found it difficult to rest. As such, I worried about the timing and frequency of her medications. I also agonized about Heather's health. Would her cancer worsen and, if so, where? Was my family keeping the truth from me? There were nights when I could see a red circle on the ceiling over my bed. Yes, it was actually there and, at times in my drugged-up state, reminded me of the Japanese Zero model plane I built when I was a young boy at my grandmother's home. At age 7 or 8, I had quite a collection of WWII fighter plane models. When I mentioned the red circle by phone to my brother,

Scott, I'm sure that he thought I was losing it. At times, he may have been correct!

During the day, I'd try to read. However, as I became weaker, that became more difficult. I studied everything I could regarding my "situation"; I even watched a heart transplant on-line! I enjoyed meeting with the "Fellows" – bright young doctors who seemed fascinated with my career.* I got to know some well and, with a few, still correspond today. I learned where they went to school, what they liked and, save medicine, how little many knew about life. That's when/where I mentored those young docs. The latter, thinking me noetic and intrigued by my global experiences, returned to my room regularly for coffee and "Professor Cunha's tutorials".

The CCU nurses were calm, compassionate, competent and considerate. They treated Mary and me very respectfully. Occasionally, they even worked around Mary's cot so that she might rest a bit more. Among those nurses, I adored several and respected all. In addition to their tender competence, one of the senior nurses (probably to curtail my singing) burned for me some beautiful opera tapes. When my Swan was off, my favorite male nurse would shave me very carefully in areas remote from where

---

*   As an international banker, consultant and volunteer, I had worked in over 50
      countries.

my Swan had been. A couple of my other favorite nurses brought me delicious (doctor-approved/low sodium) cookies. The best, however, was a Christmas gift from one of my all-time favorite nurses. As Christmas approached, and when I was too weak to read any more, that nurse gave me a beautiful Christmas bookmark. I promised her that, every year for the rest of my life, her bookmark would adorn my Christmas tree. The following quote on the bookmark was especially timely and poignant: "For I know the plans I have for you", declares the Lord. "Plans to prosper you and not to harm you. Plans to give you hope and a future". (Jeremiah 29:11)

I should also mention a P.A. who was exceptional in providing me with both insightful care and useful medical information. That P.A. was one of the brightest individuals in the CCU. More importantly, he took the time to draw detailed medical illustrations for me – hence explaining patiently some of what I was undergoing. I don't know if he will take my advice, but I hope that my special P.A. will attend medical school. He would make an extraordinary doctor: skill juxtaposed by a blend of caring, patience and humility.

At night, my five nurses of Indian heritage would take turns talking and praying with me. All were extremely

religious and, through their Christian faith, seemed to believe fervently that I "would make it to the other side".
Thankfully, these friends were on-board Halloween night
(10/31/13) when it seemed that I was having a heart attack.

That frightful Halloween night, one of my nurses of
Indian descent stayed with me constantly. As she held my
hand, we prayed together softly. We asked our Holy Mother
to give me more time – even if only a few more days.
Since "my Mary" was trick or treating with Jennifer's kids
in Roswell, Georgia, she was not with me when this epi-
sode began. However, when my condition seemed grave,
that nurse called Mary and told her that I "missed her".
Quite tactfully, she added "please drive carefully but come
quickly". On that inauspicious night, Mary saw me at, to
date, the worst I had ever been. Remarkably, after hours
of horrible chest pains, nitroglycerine, prayers, and positive thinking, the attending cardiac doctor was able to control my arrhythmias, stabilize my pounding heart, manage
my elevated blood pressure and, gradually, cause my chest
pains to subside. I simply refused to die that night; after all,
it was one day after my daughter, Jennifer's 40th birthday.
Obviously, on that dark night, providence was on my side.

Mary stayed in-touch with family and friends. As the
cornucopia of get-well cards arrived, she patiently read

them to me. I never thought that I had so many friends. Many days Mary and I would talk about the future. We especially reveled in planning special trips with our grandkids. These conversations prompted me to make an active/ future (_not_ "*bucket*") list of things to do when I had a new heart. Mary was very positive and always believed that the time would come and the Red Phone would ring for me. Then, together, we would finally enjoy our golden years. It had been six long years of sickness, pain and doctors – including, on three occasions, Mary's *critical* hospitalizations. As Mary and I prayed together for contentment and strength, she would grasp my hand tightly (as it trembled from my meds.) and tell me that all would be well. I believed her and, moreover, having climbed some sizable mountains in my life (both personally and professionally), I sensed that, down the road, there was at least *one candle* still illuminated for me. I reasoned that the greatest distance in life is what's between my ears. Indeed, in that area of my brain, I felt strong. I knew that, no matter how awful, I could take whatever was thrown at me. Despite my pain and lassitude, I was resolute and knew in my mind and soul that I would win this battle. *I would not surrender*!

As I tried to make the best of a bad situation, Mary reminded me of the things left undone (including writing this book), and of the thousands of people (especially in less developed countries) who had benefited from my financial advice, consulting and volunteer work. Mary emphasized the distances I had traveled in my life, the adversity I had conquered and the peaks I had assaulted. We smiled together as we thought about our daughters: their fine educations, solid marriages and, of course, our five beautiful and bright grandchildren. Mary helped groom me when family or friends were expected to visit me in my tiny hospital room and, afterwards, reminded me how I "lit up" when I talked with people – especially our grandkids.

As with my proactive advocacy for her (sometimes critical) hospitalizations over the past six years, Mary also provided me with both solid "bench strength" and positive oversight regarding my care. Albeit sometimes upset herself (justifiably from worry, pain, exhaustion, stress, etc.), Mary accepted my occasional rage at life and helped me confront better my anxious dreams. Together, occasionally cuddled up in my bed (reluctantly allowed by my nurses!), we would listen to our favorite song: Kenny Rogers' "Through The Years".

The days passed very slowly. There were always more tests. To measure my antibodies for compatibility, even the CDC got involved. After all, I had traveled to some "strange" places and the donor's heart and mine would have to be compatible. I missed Halloween with my grandkids and Thanksgiving at my cousin Keith's house. Thanksgiving with my cousins, Keith and his wife, Cathy, and their large family was always a feast filled with love, gratitude and fun.

By late November, my body ached with pain. Occasionally, I struggled to fight back tears of desperation. However, fear was <u>never</u> an issue; rather, my biggest distractions were chronic discomfort, impatience, boredom and agonizing concerns about my family. Although I worried most about Heather and Mary's health, my head often throbbed from the stress I perceived on Jennifer's family. It was 35 miles each way from Jennifer's home to EUH. Although I was grateful for Jennifer's frequent visits, I knew that they involved juggling her active family's schedules and navigating through/around Atlanta's horrible traffic.

Even though the weather had become very cold, I craved more than ever fresh air. Sensing this, one of my favorite "Fellows", a kind man of Ukrainian roots, smuggled me out of my room for a walk. Enabled by a wheelchair and covered with blankets, we clandestinely traversed the hospital's halls and, God bless him, he took me outside the main entrance for about 5 minutes. The cold air was, in a positive sense, breathtaking and, as I rejoiced, I greeted everyone who I could see with a broad smile and a "Merry Christmas". When I returned to my room, the Nursing Director was upset with my Fellow/Doctor – that is until she saw us laughing boisterously together. Although that bright, talented and caring man has moved away from Atlanta, I still try to stay in-touch with him.

I yearned to be home for Christmas. Each morning, as a weak palliative, I would sing (naturally off-key) – "I'll be home for Christmas". I was very weak, had lost almost 15 pounds and, as I sat-up to sing, it was quite difficult. Indeed, my voice had become mellifluous, dull and weak. Nevertheless, to me, I sounded like Bing Crosby – and that's what mattered! I was especially delighted when some of my nurses, techs. and/or patients would join me in song. What a unique and unforgettable chorus!

CHAPTER VII:

December

"The things that we love tell us what we are"

—St. Thomas Aquinas

For Christmas, my family decorated CCU-409 beautifully. There were two small Christmas trees donated by friends, a few lights and various Christmas ornaments. Nevertheless, by mid-December, I was extremely weak, debilitated and colorless. I was "circling the drain" between life and death!

On December 16th, at around 9:00 am, I was thrilled to receive a call from Cardinal Dolan, Archbishop of New York. When he called, I was in an inverted position being tested for fluid levels. (The docs. called that procedure a "Wedge"; I referred to it as my daily "Wedgie".)

Hyperventilating due to my awkward position and over-all weakness, I still took the call. Hearing my challenged respiration, His Eminence remarked "that it was most unusual (for him) to be speaking to someone breathing heavily on the other end of a phone". We both laughed and I told him how much I have always enjoyed Irish humor. We spoke about my critical condition and, together, we prayed. His Eminence also mentioned that I would be included in the congregation's prayers at Christmas Eve's Midnight Mass at St. Patrick's Cathedral.

Within an hour of Cardinal Dolan's call, I received an unscheduled visit from Father Morrow, a Catholic Priest from a local parish near EUH. Father Morrow (also of Irish Heritage) told me that he had been asked to visit me, hear my confession and bless me with the Last Rights of the Catholic Church. I was stunned by both Father Morrow's sudden appearance and his unset-tling message. I knew I was "fading", but what else did Father Morrow know? Nevertheless, before proceeding I asked Father Morrow if he intended to stay for dinner. When he seemed puzzled by my question, I told him (in jest) that "my confession could take a while"! We both laughed boisterously and I embraced him as only some-one might do on the edge of life. When Father Morrow departed, I told Mary that the Last Rights did not upset me; however, confessing to cheating once a little on my taxes was most disconcerting!

The day after the call from Cardinal Dolan and Father Morrow's visit, I received an e-mail from Notre Dame's Representative in Atlanta. She told me that prayers at the Grotto and at Sunday Mass for me continued at Notre Dame. I thanked her, mentioned that I was most grateful and added "I'll always love Notre Dame".

My daughter, Heather, and her family flew down from New York City to spend a week with Mary and me at Christmas. It was wonderful to have Heather, Christopher, Alexander and William close-by for this most special holiday. Of course, Jennifer, Heith, Micah, Olivia and Emory had been there regularly. But now we were all together for what might be my last Christmas. Each day for over a week my daughters and their families took turns visiting me in small groups. My doctors and nurses, sensing my sheer joy, simply closed the door to my room and let us enjoy each other. While the grandchildren played games, read stories and colored in their Christmas books, the adults reminisced about a lifetime of our family's special memories. With help from my daughters, the grandchildren often brought me a few healthy, but delicious, Christmas cookies and some hand-made/glittery cards and posters and/or short stories which each had made for me. All were heart-warming and so beautiful!

Christmas Eve and Christmas Day, my entire/immediate family visited. Both days, in between my naps, we celebrated all day. Also with us were my brother, Scott, and his wife, Melissa. Scott is 14 years younger than me. He lives in Staten Island, N.Y. and, absent children of his own, has been a caring and loving uncle to my daughters. As a child, he, too, had to contend with our always doltish, bilious and extremely selfish mother. Our Christmases with Irene (our mother) were dismal, devoid of gifts, absent church and, horribly, often featured my mother caterwauling about something trivial and unimportant. Perhaps, because of my childhood history, Mary and I have always gone overboard with our children and grandchildren at Christmas. Thus, CCU 409 had abundant Christmas presents for everyone and gala seasonal decorations everywhere!

On Christmas Day we sang Christmas carols, opened presents and rejoiced! I was even allowed to enjoy some unique Christmas treats. Without any interruptions, the entire floor of the CCU let us celebrate. However, as the day progressed, I grew increasingly weary. As I closed my eyes to rest, I asked my brother solemnly to "promise me he'd help take care of Mary". I was unafraid of dying; after all

"I had lived a life that was full and traveled each and every highway".* Rather, I was worried about my Mary! I was worn-out, drugged-up and quite sad as my family would soon leave. I was already in my third month of waiting and, strangely, in 2013 heart transplants at EUH were way below the average number. Most importantly, however, I never lost hope! After all, I thought, for those of us waiting for the miracle of a new heart, the Red Phone's chimes were long overdue! Appendix B depicts my family and me on Christmas Day 2013.

---

*   From Frank Sinatra's song (written by Paul Anka)...."*My Way*".

CHAPTER VIII:
"Cunha's A Go"

"Believe you can and you're halfway there"

—*Theodore Roosevelt*

December 31st, 2013 was the coldest day of the year. It opened as any other day: a light breakfast, followed by watching Fox News and, around noon, a boring lunch. I recall struggling to concentrate on some newspapers which friends had brought for me. As my sheets and linens were changed (as they were everyday), I sat on a chair near my bed and conversed with whomever came into my room. Mary was with me all day until about 2:00 pm.

Since it was New Year's Eve, Mary left to return home for more of her prescriptions, to acquire some fresh clothing and, at my encouragement, to visit a salon to enjoy a haircut and styling. Additionally, Mary had decided to pick-up some "innocent" champagne and permissible snacks for us to celebrate the New Year. However, later that afternoon, everything on that day – and in my life – would change dramatically!

At 4:15 pm, as I was peddling hesitatingly on an exercise bike (seated in a special chair so that I would not fall), a young nurse with whom I was unfamiliar until that day entered my room shaking. As she did, I could see a juxtaposing strange excitement among a few nurses at the nurses' station. I stopped peddling and, quivering, that angelic nurse told me that there might be a match for me tonight. Barely breathing and shaking from excitement, I asked her to say it again. She did, but advised me that it would take a few more hours to be certain. I immediately called Mary, my daughters and brother. I later learned that on every "break" for the rest of her shift that caring nurse had prayed for me in the hospital's chapel.

While waiting for my wife to return, I sat in disbelief in my bed. I prayed that the news would not have been premature, and that this night I would, indeed, see my nightmare end. After 70 hard days, could my "impossible dream" now be imminent?

Meanwhile, after picking-up her medications and fresh clothes, Mary received my frantic call at her hair salon. Despite being only half finished, she told her beautician to hurry up because she needed to return to the hospital for her husband "to receive a new heart"!

Mary returned to my room at approximately 5:15 pm. By then, the doctors and nurses had already begun the process of preparing me for a possible heart transplant. As Mary and I stared at each other emotionally, volumes of blood were being taken to be used for possible transfusion. Despite all of the sudden hectic activity, we remained calm in order not to be disappointed if the match alert had been premature.

At precisely 7:17 pm, three hours and two minutes after first receiving the news that a heart may be on its way to me, the cardiac doctor on-call entered my room and showed me a text message from the surgeons. It simply read: *"Cunha's a go"!* The harvest team and surgeons had confirmed that the match was solid and, as soon as possible, my heart transplant would commence. As my young nurse wept, she informed me that "this would be her first". I responded "me too"! My main cardiac doctor called me with congratulations and I told him that, finally, I would see him "on the other side". Many of the nurses entered my room and, with Mary and me, prayed for this "miracle". At last, the Red Phone had rung for me! I hugged Mary with all the strength I could muster. She called our daughters, my brother, her sister and brother and a few close friends. Our feelings were indescribable!

CHAPTER IX:
New Year's Day

"Cometh the hour, cometh the man"

—Cliff Gladwin

Because of heavy transplant/surgical demands all day on New Year's Eve, I learned later that the surgeons were required to have rest and recovery time before operating on some others and me. Consequently, the harvest team had to keep my donor alive artificially for several hours longer until early morning on New Year's Day. At around 9:00 pm on New Year's Eve I was given anti-anxiety and sleep medications to help me relax and remain calm through an incredible night.

The medications did little to make me sleepy; I was simply too excited! Mary and I talked non-stop and, as we cuddled on my hospital bed, watched television as the New Year arrived around the world. The nurses brought sparkling cider and snacks around – but, for me, they were off limits because of my impending surgery. Around midnight, after many deep hugs and tender kisses, Mary and I finally slept for a couple of hours.

On New Year's Day 2014 at 3:00 am, the nurses woke us for my final preparations. By then my daughter, Jennifer and her husband had arrived from their home in Roswell, GA. They were delayed a few hours as they had to make arrangements for the care of their children – Micah, Olivia and Emory. Mary advised me again that, as soon as possible, Heather would be flying down from NYC and be joining her, Jennifer and Heith in a waiting area proximate to the OR. Mary also mentioned that, unfortunately, my brother, Scott, was very sick and could not make the trip. However, she had promised to keep him posted. I overheard the nurses tell Mary that the operation would take approximately 10 hours followed by 2 or 3 more hours in recovery. Nevertheless, Mary was comforted in knowing that every couple of hours while I was in surgery a doctor or nurse would leave the OR to visit her in the waiting room with an update/ progress report.

Just before I was taken to the OR, Mary and I learned from a nurse that neither of the two surgeons who had been scheduled for my surgery would be available. Already that night, they had accumulated too many hours in surgery. Therefore, my principal surgeon would be a doctor from St. Joseph's Hospital, an EUH affiliate. That was an important detail, and Mary and I should have met the St. Joseph's surgeon and been briefed by him <u>before</u> I headed down the hall to the OR.[*]

As I left the CCU, I waived to the wonderful nurses who were standing by to see me depart for the OR. With tears in my eyes, I told them that I would not see them again in the CCU. Indeed, my arduous CCU wait was finished! Yet, despite the imminent removal of my heart (and possible death), my mind rejoiced in the fact that, finally, there would be an end to the agonizing uncertainty of the past 70 days. Although I believed in my soul that this approaching miracle would be successful, I still told those nursing angels that – in one place or another – I would see them on "the other side". By that I meant, I'd either see them soon in the ICU or, if not, eventually in God's heaven!

It was about 4:00 am on January 1, 2014 (New Year's Day) as I traveled to the OR. Along the way, I recall singing

---

[*]   As mentioned in an earlier chapter, while in the CCU I had asked to meet one – if not both – of the surgeons slated eventually to do my heart transplant. For any surgery, that's quite normal. Strangely, however, I met neither of those surgeons nor the one charged with saving my life on New Year's Day. I only met the latter in the OR just before my heart transplant surgery. A supportive, informative and kind meeting beforehand would have been very comforting and reassuring to my wife and me.

passionately "The Impossible Dream". Indeed it was! I was about to beat the unbeatable foe! More importantly, I hugged and kissed Mary, Jennifer and Heith, told them I loved them and asked them to deliver the same message to Heather, Christopher, Scott and all my grandchildren.

The lights in the OR were blinding. There must have been 20 or more people in sight. Gingerly, I was taken face-up from my stretcher to the operating table. My hands were tied down as if to be crucified and, with sanctity, everyone in the room (including me) held hands and we prayed together. We prayed for the donor, his family, the doctors, nurses and me. What a surreal moment! Simultaneously, in my soon to be removed heart, I also prayed for my wife, children and grandchildren. I asked the Lord to protect them and give them strength and courage. Before losing consciousness, I recall distinctly thanking the doctor for his skill and pleading with him "not to screw-up my brain".

CHAPTER X:
"The Other Side"

"Tears come from the heart and not from the brain"

—Leonardo da Vinci

I first heard of "the other side" when I arrived in CCU-409. The message echoed by the nurses was "we need to get you to the other side"! Initially, that phrase stunned me as I interpreted it ominously. However, I soon learned that "the other side" was where I wanted to be. It was the special ICU <u>after</u> a heart transplant. Before every weekend in CCU-409, I recall wishing my principal nurses a good weekend and adding that, on Monday, I hoped to see them on the other side.

When I arrived in the ICU, I was unaware of anything. However, later my wife told me that when I arrived I "looked dead". In surgery my body temperature had been dropped precipitously – hence, according to Mary, my gray-like appearance. I was intubated and, everywhere, had tubes, catheters, Ivs, etc. in or extending from my body. I also had two large Argyle Drains inserted in my chest; these were to drain excess blood which remained in my chest. In addition, I had metallic-like wires (temporary pacing electrodes) above the right Argyle Drain. Those wires were intended to pace my heart at 110 beats a minute to increase blood flow. Those wires could also be used, if necessary, to shock my heart as, for instance, a defibrillator might. Since there was no longer a need, my pacemaker and defibrillator had been removed in surgery. Albeit very sick, critical and fragile, *I was alive!*

I was in and out of consciousness for about 1 ½ days. Then, rather abruptly, I recall awakening and moved to tears when I saw my family close by my side. Appendix C depicts Mary with me when I first legitimately woke up. I was confused, very cold and in pain. To mitigate my consternation, one of my nurses told me that the meds. being administered to me would help me with the pain. However, he added it was quite normal to feel disoriented, tremulous and extremely emotional. My God, I said to myself, I just survived a heart transplant! Although I was still intubated, I asked my nurses for a pad on which to write. I needed to know if my mind was still functioning.

Upon entering the ICU, I had two nurses in my room at all times. Sometimes, when I was coherent, having two nurses so close became annoying. Yet, I recognized that they were extremely dedicated to my care. Very kindly, they responded immediately to my requests for a writing pad and more blankets. While still intubated, the pad would allow me to write notes, ask questions and, after all, begin reassuring myself that the surgeons had not damaged my brain.

Although shaking profusely, I recall scribbling illegibly: "am I alive"?; "can my family stay with me"?; and "what day is it"? As every inch of my body hurt, I tried to write about my pain levels (10+). Scrawling on my pad, I asked to be extubated, but was informed that that would be denied until the docs. were certain that I could breathe on my own. After several attempts to determine if my brain was OK, my nurses understood and gave me a big smile and a thumbs-up.

I recognized Mary, Jennifer, Heather and Heith from the time I began to regain consciousness. Once awake, I held my daughters and wife's hands with tears streaming from my eyes. Without words, and with my eyes only, I tried to express my love for them and gratitude for this miracle. In turn, they encouraged me to try to rest. Of course, night or day, sleep was difficult. After all, my body was in turmoil! However, adding to my sleeplessness was, incredibly, the fact that my room also served as the nurses' supply closet. In addition to non-stop vigilance over me, the nurses interrupted my brief moments of rest by opening and closing that damn closet! After 2 days, when I was extubated and finally able to speak, I began to protest both the continual noise from the medical equipment (i.e., constant beeping) and the nurses' never ending slamming of the squeaky supply/ closet doors. Quite unkindly one of my nurses of Central or Eastern Europe descent actually reprimanded me for getting annoyed. For two nights that nurse had been unpleasant, agitated and seemingly upset about everything. Therefore, when she asked what I had done for a living, I responded "have you ever heard of the CIA" (clever, but untrue!).

To calm me, a kind young nurse came into my room with a mirror. She asked me to look at the mirror. Although uncaring about my caveman-like appearance, I indulged this sweet nurse. I couldn't believe what I saw! My lips were red and my face had a healthy-looking glow. It was the first time in many months that I didn't look pale and very sickly. Since the nurse simultaneously checked my heart with her stethoscope, my daughter, Heather, suggested that she allow me to listen as well. Since I was already curious about this new/distinct pounding in my chest, I took the stethoscope and listened to my new heart. What clear and supernatural sounds! My new heart was working, the beats strong and the rhythms synchronized. *I had reached my impossible dream!; I had survived my long, painful quest for a new heart*!

Once I saw Mary's cell phone, I asked her immediately to dial-up a few close friends — Dick King, Jim Long and Ira Kent. In tears and in a very faint/quivering voice, I told each "I have a new heart". I added, "gentlemen – I'm still here"! Later, after I rested, I called three other close friends: Bob Schlegel, Ken Moll and Richard Dubbs.

The ICU is vastly different from the CCU. The former is always very somber; the latter is designed to keep the patient reasonably comfortable during an agonizing wait for a heart. The CCU is usually a long, tough, debilitating stretch; typically, the ICU must treat critically ill patients (transplanted or otherwise) for a few days. Every minute in the ICU was perniciously serious. While the nurses in the CCU were generally approachable, the nurses in the ICU seemed aloof. Some ICU nurses were cantankerous and seemed unhappy. From those caring for me, I yearned most for a tender smile. When I insisted that my immediate family stay with me on the night I awoke, they were advised stridently that their visitation limits must be brief. Thankfully, as I improved, the ICU "commander" softened significantly and permitted more flexible visitation for my family. But, understandably, others had to respect the visitation protocols. Namely, zero tolerance for visitors other than my immediate family.

For instance, when my CCU nurse on New Year's Eve (recall, my "first time" nurse) came to visit me (with her entire family and with a huge bowl of fruit), she was instructed by the ICU nurses to leave. However, later that day, I was very pleased that at least she was allowed to leave that delicious fruit! Away from the ICU, Mary and my daughters did spend some time with that nurse and her gracious family. They expressed our family's gratitude for their timely prayers on New Year's Eve and for their subsequent thoughtfulness. I will always remember that nurse's devotion to my family and me!

On my fourth day in the ICU, I was instructed to walk. Recoiling in disbelief, three nurses ordered me "up"! As they carefully took my head, torso, legs and feet, I rose next to my bed. Attached to me was a trail of medical tubes, devices, Ivs, a Swan, instruments, drains, catheters, etc. A walker and a seat belt apparatus helped me get stable enough to stand. I was in pain, extremely weak, shaky, sleep-deprived, drugged-up and, naturally, very anxious about falling. Nevertheless, on that glorious day, I smiled and, feeling as if I was about to conquer Mt. Everest, took two "laps" around the ICU. (That powerful photo is on the front cover of this book.)

When I returned from my "walk", one of my transplant surgeons (albeit not the primary surgeon) was there to greet me. He was a serious man often of few words. He asked me how I was doing and advised me that my heart was young, healthy, strong and a "perfect fit". He added that when positioned in my chest and blood started flowing, the heart only needed one "tap" to start beating in its new home. That, according to my doctor, was a very good sign. Humorously, I asked him for a "warranty on my new heart". He replied, "there are no warranties in life and death". He added that "if I'd like, he could put the old one back"! We both smiled and I stated clearly – "no thanks, I'll keep my new engine"!

On my fourth day in the ICU, I called Cardinal Dolan. He had already heard the "good news" from my daughter, Heather. His Eminence and I rejoiced at God's miraculous gift and, quietly, he led me in prayer. I asked His Eminence "why it had taken so long"?; "was he losing his touch"? When Cardinal Dolan asked me what I meant, I replied that, after all, we had spoken on December 16th and here it was January 4th! Why had it taken him so long to persuade God to help me? We laughed together and His Eminence asked me to visit him at St. Patrick's Cathedral. He added that he'd like to hear my "story".

The last thing which needed to be done before I could leave the ICU for "The Floor" was to remove the Swan in my neck.

Ordinarily, the Swan removal is straightforward and not difficult to accomplish. First the stitches holding the Swan in-place are removed. Then, gently, the area disinfected and, after the Swan is removed, the wounds closed. With me, however, it wasn't that easy!

The wounds began to bleed profusely with blood flowing heavily from the gash in my neck. Since the latter opened deeply into my neck, there were some immediate concerns. Although the senior nurse handling my Swan removal didn't panic, as blood soaked my neck, chest, back, abdomen, groin, linens and floor, she called for support from another senior nurse. When I inquired about getting an M.D. involved, both nurses said they had it under control. Nevertheless, the thought occurred to me that – after surviving a long wait for a heart and a heart transplant – might I now die from bleeding to death? Could my new heart handle the sudden drop in blood pressure? The feeling of blood pouring all over me was alarming, but I tried to rationalize that I couldn't be in a better place for emergent care. Indeed, the nurses calmed the bloody storm and, with pressure, bandages, etc. were finally able (after about 15 minutes) to stop the bleeding. What a relief from a rather disquieting situation!

Keys to my ICU strength were my faith and family's support. Mary, Jennifer and Heather were there round-the-clock. Heith was also there regularly. My Roswell grandchildren, Micah, Olivia and Emory, were permitted to visit once. Albeit brief, their visit was very inspirational. My grandsons in Old Greenwich, CT, Alexander and William, conveyed "messages" (Alexander directly and William, given his age, vicariously). There, too, those tidings gave me strength and hope. They, as well as the calls from my son-in-law, Christopher, brother, Scott, and sisters-in-law, Melissa and Joan, encouraged me that I would soon "nose up". They made me believe that I would see blue skies again! I will always be profoundly grateful for my family's love and support on The Other Side. Appendix D is a photo of my daughters and me on my fourth day in the ICU.

After 5 days in the ICU, I was transferred to "The

Floor". Still attached were all the paraphernalia needed to survive. However, for the first time in almost three months, neither a Swan nor a Picc Line remained. I felt that my move to the Floor represented real progress in my efforts finally to go home.

CHAPTER XI:
"The Floor"

"Attitude is the little thing that makes a big difference"

—Winston Churchill

The Floor is a hospital zone directly adjacent to the ICU. It serves as the place where heart transplant patients (among others) who are deemed well enough to transition from the ICU reside after surgery. Nurses are attentive, but not to the extent in either the CCU or, certainly, the ICU. The Floor was my next step in terms of eventually exiting the hospital.

Although some of my nurses on the Floor were helpful, one was truly outstanding. That lady, born in Africa (don't recall the country) and an avid runner, was the model of what all nurses should be. She resembled some of my best CCU nurses. She patiently and thoroughly explained this stage of my care. I will never forget this extraordinary lady's professionalism, kindness, patience and special care.

Shortly after I arrived, a large man appeared in my room. He was there to remove the electrode/wire device from my chest. Deemed no longer necessary, this device could now be removed and this man (a P.A.) had the job of pulling it out of my chest. Mary and I were very concerned at the time because we had witnessed a patient return to the ICU in critical condition because of an indelicate withdrawal of that device. The electrode's removal had critically injured the man's new heart. Nevertheless, it was time for my electrodes to be extracted. Therefore, as with most things for the past several months, I merely surrendered to fate. Whereas a modicum of instructions, expectations, etc. might have been considerate, this bilious P.A. simply approached my bed and, gripping the electrode firmly, withdrew it from my chest. When I objected to not having fair warning, he walked away and, nonchalantly, said "you'll be fine". A few days later I would suffer through another encounter with this boorish man.

Every day, multiple times a day, a nurse would enter my room and announce that another blood and/or lung capacity test, weight check, insulin check, etc. must be done immediately. Although I didn't have diabetes, the sudden introduction and potency of my meds. sometimes caused diabetic symptoms in some heart transplant patients. If my numbers were off, insulin would be administered. Nevertheless, day or night, I always told the nurses "how great it was to *see* them". However, I learned that my reaction was unique. At night, many patients griped about constant nursing and tech. interruptions. Moreover, quite early on some mornings, some doctors would enter rooms, turn on *all* the lights and bellow *good morning*! Those docs., some in puberty a decade ago, seemed insensitive to the fact that every two hours all night long some nurse and/or tech. had arrived in my room to check vitals, deliver meds., draw blood, etc. In fact, one night at 4:00 a.m., Mary and I were startled by a tech. who, after dragging a device noisily into my room (immediately recognized as a scale!), asked me to get out of bed so that she could weigh me. God knows why that "procedure" couldn't have been combined with my 6:00 am wake-up call for meds. Nevertheless, some early bird doctors' cacophonous early morning arrivals upset Mary and me the most. On one morning, in particular, the young doctor's morning "announcement" was accompanied by her remarkable lack of preparation before entering my room.

As the doctor began to probe as to how I was, it became obvious that she was unprepared for that 6:00 am morning visit. When I inquired if she had read my file, the doctor stated dismissively that, since she had been on vacation for two weeks, she was "behind" with her patients. She wanted an update from me as to "what was going on". I was outraged; how could she arrive in my room (or any room) unprepared? As Mary and I expressed our deep concerns about the doctor's demeanor, the electrode man entered my room to inquire as to "our problem". Now here I was 9 days out from a heart transplant and this ribald lad decided to reprimand Mary and me for our reproach to the young doctor. Naturally, too weak to fight back (or even to get a word in!), we simply let it go. However, at least now for posterity, neither that bumptious doc. nor that obnoxious P.A. have been overlooked for their extraordinarily callous and unprofessional behavior.

The next interlude on the Floor was removing a "sensitive" catheter. It happened quickly and, thankfully, not by the electrode guy. Save a wince (mine, not my nurse's!), it was welcome relief for me. The catheter's existence had been very awkward and most unpleasant.

While all this was happening, some of my CCU nurses began appearing outside my room. When I was encumbered by Floor medical personnel, my Floor nurses had my CCU nurses wait outside my room to see me. However, as they entered one at a time, my emotions took over and, as I hugged some of these wonderful people, the tears flowed as if a faucet had been turned-on. Over 15 of my CCU nurses visited me and, with each, I shared a huge smile. It was a triumphantly moving experience which I will never forget and savor forever.

The final step in my Floor stay was the removal of the two large Argyle Drains. To that, I was not looking forward. Two former heart transplant recipients who very kindly visited me regularly in the CCU, mentioned their "out-of-body experiences" when their drains were removed. By the way, those two heart transplant recipients and their wives are truly wonderful examples of paying it forward. They are extraordinarily generous people to whom I am indebted for their kind advice and timely meetings with Mary and me.

Returning to the drains, once again my philosophy was just to let it happen. Although I expected an M.D. to be on-board to wrench the drains from my chest, it turned out to be my favorite Floor nurse. As she approached me confidently to begin the extraction, I jokingly asked her if she was "qualified". Respectfully, she replied that, "without incident", she had done this many times. Very patiently, my nurse asked me to sit-up, take a deep breath and relax. She then grabbed hold of both drains simultaneously and instructed me to exhale deliberately. Anxiously, I then watched this talented/slight of physique nurse uproot the drains from my body. My feelings as the drains left my chest were, indeed, akin to a most bizarre experience. It felt as if my insides had suddenly been vacated. My nurse then asked me to lay on my back for at least two hours to avoid any complications. I obliged and, with Mary now at my side, fell asleep. Regrettably, for us both, Mary was disallowed from being in my room during any of the aforementioned Floor procedures. (The same strict protocols applied when I was in the CCU and ICU.)

Each day on the Floor, I pressed for a bowel movement. I hadn't had relief since New Year's Eve! In addition to my post-op. pains everywhere, my abdomen and back ached from my body or mind's disinclination to strain. The nurses gave me the usual remedies, but success was not forthcoming. Each day, I called the dining "concierge" pleading for prune juice. However, since my diet was carefully monitored, I was usually informed that this item would have to be considered my *one* "daily snack". Struggling to avoid painful/unrestrained laughter, I simply replied: "of course... and please hurry up since it's desperately needed to help promote an important event!"

January 2014, the weather in Atlanta was the coldest in history. My room on the Floor in the hospital's old section faced the wind and, with the temperature hovering around 6 degrees, my room was <u>extremely</u> cold. When EUH's compassionate CEO visited me to see how I was doing, he noticed that – even with four blankets – I was shivering. He immediately asked a tech. nearby to go to his office and retrieve his personal space heater. What a kind thing to do; it was one of several exceptionally sensitive acts attributable to this fine man during my stay at EUH.

By the fifth day on the Floor, albeit gingerly and with help, I was able to stand and walk. Although hesitatingly, my docs. began to suggest that I should leave for Mason House. When Mary and I pushed back (as we both felt that it was much too soon), my doctors advised us that flu was becoming epidemic in the hospital and, as such, I was extremely vulnerable. Indeed, infections are main contributors to death after heart transplants. Therefore, my always cautious docs. felt it would be best if I could find a safe harbor as soon as possible. Not expecting this turn of events, Mary and I scrambled to begin the process of assembling the items on which we had survived for almost three months. As Mary was returning home with some of what we had accumulated, I was making calls to secure our stay at Mason House, a transition facility near the hospital. Mind you, all this was occurring about ten days after a heart transplant! With me barely standing and on the phone, my brother, Scott, and sister-in-law, Melissa, entered my room.

An understatement would be to say that Scott and Melissa were shocked to see me upright. Truth be told, every part of me was rebelling violently as my body tried to cast off this new object by which it had been invaded. Also, my meds. were causing tumultuous reactions (or, in some instances, inactions) in some very unpleasant ways. Nevertheless, seeing Scott and Melissa was joyful and, thankfully it seemed, Scott had recovered from the nasty flu which had plagued him since Christmas.

The last step before leaving the Floor was to receive final instructions on my medications. The complexity of those meds. cannot be minimized. In my room, EUH's chief pharmacist conveyed the life or death precision with which the cornucopia of my meds. must be taken. Graphs and charts displayed the seriousness of not being careful. The first year, for instance, would be the most complicated, difficult and *riskiest*. If my heart transplant was not meant to be, deadly rejection was most likely in the first 6-12 months.

As Mary took careful notes, I tried to sort the drug details into my mind's "buckets" for storage and recall. Within hours, I received an enormous bag full of drugs and related paraphernalia. It was overwhelming, but critically important. On the positive side, my pharmacist advised me that, in time (perhaps in 6 months), my prednisone dosage might be tapered. However, all other meds., including a few powerful anti-rejection drugs, would probably not be tapered for at least 18 months. Noteworthy, however, I would be taking anti-rejection meds. for the rest of my life. I listened carefully as I was told that, at least initially, the side-effects of many medications (some individually, some in concert with others) could be painful, harsh, disorienting and, sometimes, disabling. But, after all, I was breathing and vertical! As Mary and I left the Floor (she walking, me riding in a wheelchair), we waved a heartfelt good-bye to EUH. In return, some of the nurses clapped, gave me high fives and wished me a belated Happy Birthday (i.e., January 1st). We were off to Mason House.

CHAPTER XII:
Mason House

Mason House is a private retreat on the Emory University campus. Donated by Carlos Mason[*] and his wife, Marguerite, it offers temporary/transitional housing for organ transplant recipients. Mason House serves as a temporary home-away-from home – hence allowing patients to be away from the hospital but close enough to feel secure should they need medical assistance quickly.

For most Mason House was the first time away from the CCU or ICU in many months. Naturally, recipients are unsure of what they can do on their own and uncomfortable without the hospital's umbrella of instantaneous and dedicated medical care. My initial thoughts included:

---

[*]   Carlos Mason (1873 -1955) was a successful businessman and philanthropist in Atlanta.

Will my new heart be reliable?; What should I do about the never-ending pain in every conceivable part of my body?; If needed, how long will it take to get me to my cardiac docs.?; Will my wife feel comfortable attending to me without any direct hospital support? After all, there were no doctors or nurses at Mason House. However, in an emergency, an ambulance or an escort in a golf cart would be available immediately to take me to the ER. The Mason House to ER logistics were comforting; the ER was only 5 minutes away.

Mason House is a large, elegant home set at the edge of magnificent woods and gardens. The long rear deck with many comfortable chairs overlooks an active stream. For me, even in January, it was paradise to sit briefly on the deck and, once again, appreciate nature. As I inhaled fresh (albeit cold) air, I began to realize that, seemingly, my former pre-transplant breathing concerns had disappeared. This made me smile and amazed as some old/good feelings were resurrected after 6 long years.

Mason House's first floor had a grand foyer with a winding staircase rising to the bedrooms. Naturally, there was an elevator to serve all four floors of the home. The extensive first floor parlor included a magnificent fireplace, a grand piano and several quiet areas with sofas and chairs for residents and their families to relax. After dinner, many residents gathered in the parlor to listen to a recent organ recipient play exquisitely on the piano. We all felt the glow of special companionship as soft music and tender songs filled the room. Some, including me, often sang with the music!

Elsewhere on the first floor were a few small private rooms where a resident and/or his family could chat, watch television or quietly relax. There was also a dining room with several tables and chairs, a fireplace and lovely French Door access to the deck and screened-in porch. Naturally, all areas were decorated very tastefully.

The unique kitchen was large enough for four separate work areas. Each area had a stove, oven, microwave, dishwasher and sink. Naturally, there were plenty of dishes and cookware readily available. The spacious kitchen and distinct work areas allowed each resident and his/her family to prepare their meals in a relaxed and comfortable setting. The grand kitchen also had two large refrigerators/ freezers and a deep pantry to store appropriately each resident's food.

For the first time in over three months my meals were prepared by my wife and, except for being mindful of sodium, unregulated. All residents prepared their own food

and dined when they desired. Of course, there were over-
laps in the kitchen and/or dining room, but everyone respected each other's space. I often felt, given our common
circumstances, a sense of divine companionship with these
new friends.

Occasionally, notices were placed in the main foyer to
announce common meals for all to share. Each resident,
his/her family or caretaker would make something special
from their food stocks and present it appetizingly for a
common lunch or dinner. One night, Mary brought a beautifully decorated cake just to celebrate life. Those "common" times together were magical!

The finished basement level included a workout/exer-
cise room with a large screen TV, pool table and board
games. Just to reminisce about the "old days" (i.e., before
heart failure), and to imagine a healthier future, I actually
ventured briefly into the weight room.

During our seven day stay at Mason House, residents
included 12 recent transplant recipients and their care-
givers. On the second floor there were several bedrooms.
Although some bedrooms were larger than others, each
guest had his/her own room to share with a spouse, family member or caregiver. All rooms were private and comfortable and had a full bathroom. My room was among

the smaller ones because our hospital stay was a week shorter than expected. Therefore, we were fortunate even to have a room. Nevertheless, I: *savored* the opportunity to be hospital-free and wearing normal clothes instead of hospital gowns; *embraced* my good fortune in sleeping again with my wife; *relished* the chance to be outside again in the fresh air (even in January); *marveled* at the miracle of walking (albeit very slowly) without breathing heavily; and *adored* taking showers again. (I hadn't had a shower or bath in nearly 3 months!) I hurt constantly (even my hair!) – but my mind, heart and soul were utterly joyous!

Mary catered not only to my meal and snack needs, but also oversaw my numerous and complex medications. She observed carefully my pain levels, and insisted that I rest frequently. The clothes Mary brought from home for me felt as if they were brand new. They smelled fresh and devoid of hospital scents. Those scents had been in my pores for over three months. Even today, when I return to EUH, I pick-up quickly unique hospital "patinas". Although not repugnant, those odors are to me unmistakable.

My principal complaint at Mason House was the bed shared by Mary and me. Even though it was advertised as "queen-size", it felt smaller. However, for the most part that was irrelevant as I couldn't move too much anyway. Nevertheless, my main issue with the bed was the distance from the bed to the floor; the bed was very low! That made it difficult and painful both to get-up and to relax my body enough to lay down. Each time I was faced with either dilemma, I cringed at the expectation of extra/imminent pain. Mary helped by either lifting or settling me – but, for her, that was very hard. Often, at the side of the bed, I had to assume a mendicant position in order to make it up or down. By the 5th day, I'd grown tired of sleeping on my back. Therefore, despite my doctor's orders, I decided to take a risk and, resolutely, rolled-over on my left side. As I did, I smiled to myself at this small victory!

Special treats were visits from my family and a few friends. Although Mary continued to broker all of my calls, she briefed me on the sentiments and I was always grateful for the good wishes. Additionally, my family's visits raised my spirits noticeably. Marvelously, Scott and Melissa were able to stay nearby for a few days and, when they visited, Scott always made me laugh (and, despite the added excruciating pain, in my soul it "felt" good to laugh!). It was so wonderful to be with my family in a home-like atmosphere. For Mary and me, Scott and Melissa also made some special trips to the pharmacy to reload my pain meds., pick-up bandages, gauze, food items, etc. For that and, their affection, I'm most grateful to my brother and his wife!

Jennifer and her family visited Mary and me frequently and, with them, I enjoyed unique hugs (in our family, aka "hugaroos") and some special snacks. With Heather's family in CT., we orchestrated a few Face Time conversations; they, too, included hugaroos (albeit "long distance")! Naturally, my grandchildren's remarkable cards and amazing artwork traveled with me from my decorated EUH rooms to Mason House. Those distinct and sentimental gifts – as well as the special love of my precious grandchildren – always made me extraordinarily happy!

Mason House was an amazing blessing. The staff were kind and patient. To the extent possible, I have tried to stay-in-touch with some of the guests who shared that unique time with Mary and me. Albeit briefly in my quest, I was honored to meet these people. They, as well as a few who shared my remarkable journey in the CCU, will always be my "transplant buddies"!

CHAPTER XIII:

Going Home

*"Start by doing what's necessary; then do what's possible;
and suddenly you are doing the impossible"*

—*St. Francis of Assisi*

There are no words to describe my feelings as Mary and I left Mason House. We were headed home! It had been over three months since I enjoyed my beautiful home and slept in my own bed. I was so excited that Mary had to calm me down. Because I was so vulnerable to injury (i.e., my chest, new heart, etc.), I was required to sit in the back seat of our car carefully buckled-in with my seat belt and vigilantly tucked-in with a pillow to protect my chest's vulnerability. My mind wandered as I saw sights that I hadn't seen for quite awhile. Given the heavy meds., my body shook from both post-transplant tremors and the anxiety of finally being on my way home. But I was alive and that's what mattered!

When Mary and I arrived home, I was greeted by a huge *Welcome Home* banner, balloons, smiles, joy and overwhelming excitement. My daughter, Jennifer, and her children had planned for my arrival and were there to celebrate their Dad/G-Dad's glorious homecoming. Appendix E depicts a photo taken as I arrived home on that very special day. With me were my daughter, Jennifer, and grandchildren – Micah, Olivia and Emory. My daughter, Heather, and her sons, Alexander and William, joined us by phone. Once again, my emotions took over and tears flowed from my eyes. Even for this man who prides himself on being articulate, I was speechless!

That night I slept fairly well; undoubtedly from sheer exhaustion and the absence of interruptions! My bed, of course, felt marvelous! For the first week or so I slept as much as I could. My body and mind had been through so much and were in dire need of rest and tranquility. Mary, too, spent a lot of time sleeping and resting. After all, she, too, was debilitated by our long ordeal together.

My doctors had warned me a bit about what the next year might be like. My initial reaction was that I had suffered through a 2 ½ month wait for a heart, a heart transplant, the "other side" experience, post-operation agony, countless procedures and numerous harsh meds. How bad could it be? All along my quest, even when asked directly, my doctors were circumspect about post-transplant information. The reason, I sensed, was that some patients might actually forgo a heart transplant if they knew what lay ahead. Indeed, physically, mentally, logistically (e.g., countless visits to/from EUH), etc. it would be <u>very</u> challenging. Moreover, amidst trying to recover from a heart transplant, one would have to cope with ineptly-managed and insensitive health insurance companies. Insurance issues would become <u>constant</u> (frequently redundant!) and often plagued by indifferent and careless customer service.

Each day of the first year pains in my chest and adjacent areas were accompanied by incredible pains elsewhere. Everything from my big toe to my hair (and all in-between) felt as if I had been hammered. Obviously, some pains were from my surgery; however, ancillary pains arose from my body's urgent desire to reject this new foreign object (i.e., my new heart). As I kept a daily record of my blood pressure, heart rate, temperature, etc., I also quickly discovered that my heart rate no longer increased as before because some of the nerves which control the heart were cut during surgery (e.g., the Vagus Nerve). Therefore, as a passenger in a car for instance,

I often overreacted to strange road stimuli and perceived driving threats. I also became extremely protective of my new heart. Indeed, with any close sudden movement or loud sounds by others, I would flinch and, defensively, rest both arms across my chest.

Two and one half weeks after checking out of Mason House, I was back in EUH. Concerned about the unusual rhythms in my chest, as well as the peculiar "mapping" of my blood pressure, Mary drove me to EUH. I was admitted immediately. After checking my vitals, my principal cardiac doctor suspected that my body was rejecting my new heart. Thankfully, it was not rejection – but, rather, unusual and dangerous arrhythmias. The remedies were new meds. to control the arrhythmias and gyrating blood pressure. Also, complete bed rest. At least over the week I was in the hospital, I was able to watch a (rather lopsided!) Super Bowl. I felt overwhelming relief that my heart had not been rejected. Indeed, I felt blessed at this sign that I was on the right track.

Upon returning home, I continued my isolation from family and friends. Risks of colds, infections, etc. were omnipresent! Also, my torso ached everywhere and I tired very quickly. My body simply wanted my new heart gone. To offset that natural physiological reaction, I was taking a cornucopia of immunosuppressant (i.e., anti-rejection) drugs and countless other powerful prescriptions to counter the side effects of my anti-rejection medications. Paroxysms of all shapes and forms erupted from, in and around my body and psyche. Nothing "worked" as before; everything was swollen; and my mind was tortured with bizarre thoughts, emotional/unexplainable flare-ups and peculiar "observations". Especially hard were some of the abdominal "side-effects". For those, I took every medicine imaginable but the "results" were disappointing and my guts always felt as if they were about to explode. Many of these symptoms lasted for three to four months. Among the harshest were the abdominal pains and pounding headaches. As my body convulsed, it was difficult for Mary and me to sleep. Hence, sleeplessness had a pernicious effect on my recovery and made Mary's health also deteriorate. That worried me daily! Definitely, part of my exit discussion on The Floor should have been a heads-up on some of the possible imminent challenges. To be forewarned would have been helpful and, at least for me, caused less anxiety in the months ahead. While in the CCU the focus had been to keep me alive and get me to the other side, and post-op. in the ICU my situation was critical. In fairness, however, each individual blessed with a transplant is unique. Accordingly, his/her post op. reactions and tolerances (physical and otherwise) may be quite different and vary to lesser or greater degrees.

After three months of anguish, I was happy to see spring arrive. Albeit still quite chilly, Mary took me for my first outing in almost 5 1/2 months. It was to see my grandson, Micah, play lacrosse. What a thrill and, at least for me, a *major triumph* as I ventured forth outside. Hesitatingly and freezing in the still chilly air (being personally colder than usual became part of my new reality), I walked virtually around the lacrosse field to see my dear grandson. Although the walk exhausted me, for that brief moment this 69 year-old man felt like an excited boy. My body hurt everywhere from the medications' ugly side-effects – but I was elated to be alive and outdoors near my grandson watching him play his favorite sport. Unfortunately, I was only able to watch for about 30 minutes as I felt quite cold and very tired.

After the lacrosse game, I yearned to see as soon as possible all of my very athletic and talented grandchildren participate in their favorite sports and activities. Namely: Micah - lacrosse and basketball; Olivia – volleyball and theater; Alexander – soccer and swimming; Emory – swimming and dance; and baby William – swimming and soccer. However, given risks of rejection and/or infections, all/any indoor activities (save those in a highly protected/ disinfected environment) and/or crowds would have to be avoided for at least 5-6 more months. This was an especially dangerous period as some of my drugs were being changed, tapered, adjusted, etc. Often my body literally vibrated uncontrollably from the effects of my medications. Yet, I was so grateful simply to be hungering for life!

Despite appearances to the contrary, the spring, summer and fall of 2014 continued to be very difficult for me. Although most of the time camouflaging my feelings, I required regular naps. I was always very weary. The pain and harsh meds. were still part of my life and, occasionally, my symptoms became intolerable. Mary could sense when it was especially hard for me to function. Sleeplessness, abdominal issues, headaches, disorientation and trembling continued daily. Frequent trips (i.e., at least once a week) to EUH wore Mary and me down. Adding to our stress was the difficulty at times to navigate through the complex corridors of EUH to find and arrange appointments with doctors outside the scope of cardiology. Additionally, weekly — then monthly — biopsies of my heart to determine rejection were quite painful. Regrettably, at times, the pain, inharmonious meds., lack of sleep and utter frustration all clashed and made me respond contentiously to unexpected and/or upsetting situations.

Regular heart (or myocardial) biopsies were very important. They ensured that there was not any rejection occurring. In the Cath. Lab., prone on a table, a small catheter was inserted in my neck and, using an echocardiogram, guided to my heart. The catheter has a grasping device on its end and, using that device, 4 pieces of my heart were removed for analysis. I always scheduled these biopsies on days when Mary would be able to drive and, equally important, when I could benefit from one of my favorite cardiologist's "soft hands". That doctor, an elegant lady of national prominence, always handled my biopsies deftly and in a caring manner. I feel fortunate to have benefited from her competence and conversations.

Mary, too, had doctors' appointments almost every week; she for numerous disturbing, serious and painful neurological/neurologically-based, sleep, cancer/ cancer-related and orthopedic problems. We agonized that we had been in Georgia for over 7 years and had seen virtually nothing of Atlanta and/or anything in the southeast except for highways. When we moved south, we had planned on seeing Atlanta's landmarks and cultural sites. Naturally, we had hoped to revisit interesting destinations such as Savannah, Charleston, St. Simons Island, Amelia Island, and more. Unfortunately, as time passed we gradually became out-of-the loop with friends, unable to plan ahead, sometimes melancholy in our unfulfilled retirement years, and distressed at the amount of opportunities "wasted" as we spent a disproportionate amount of time in hospitals, with doctors, submitting to tests, and coping with ongoing medical issues. Nevertheless, when I felt discouraged I needed only to reflect for a moment on my donor and his family. My donor would never again experience the joy of life and his family would always grieve at their incomprehensible loss. In turn, I was alive and my new heart offered me an opportunity to live many more years.

In 2014, we still pushed forward and, wherever possible, managed to delight in some of our grandchildren's sports activities (both boys and girls) and our granddaughters' marvelous theatrical and musical performances. Occasionally, we were able to dine with friends and, one-on-one, had special dinners just to talk with each of our grandchildren. We also adjusted our doctors' schedules to babysit from time-to-time for our daughters, sons-in-law and special grand dog, Gipper. For a few special outings, I even played 9 holes of golf. Also, occasionally, I began to review and update my notes in the hope that I might lecture again in the future at Emory and/or Notre Dame's Business Schools (respectively, Goizueta and Mendoza).

As mid-November approached, Mary and I began to look forward excitedly to being together in CT for Thanksgiving. Jennifer's family and we traveled to Old Greenwich, CT to spend a long Thanksgiving week with Heather and her family. It was the first time (albeit quite reluctantly) that my docs. allowed me to fly. The conditions were fourfold: (i) the flight would be brief and non-stop; (ii) in airports, planes, cars and any crowded areas, I would always wear a surgical/protective mask; (iii) I must be near a sophisticated major hospital (e.g., Greenwich/Yale New Haven); and (iv) I would stay indoors. Thanksgiving was very satisfying and, especially in 2014, I cherished those special days together with our whole family. As we feasted on Heather and Chris' fine Thanksgiving dinner, we thanked God wholeheartedly for our good fortune and many blessings over the past year. Appendix F is a photo of our family at Thanksgiving 2014.

A week before Christmas, the 2014 annual Dickens Dinner at our Country Club was, for me, the most spectacular since we moved to Georgia. Mary, Jennifer and her family looked happy and festive; the ladies and girls looked stunning; the men very handsome in their finest attire. We all missed Heather's family – but, reluctantly, I've come to realize that, quite fairly, our daughters must also spend holiday time with their in-laws. At the Dickens

Dinner, it was wonderful to see and talk to friends – many of whom I had not seen for quite a while. Although it was nice to hear from some friends that I looked well, my principal interest that night was to learn what had been happening in their lives.

During that enchanting near-Christmas evening, my beautiful Olivia and I sang "The Impossible Dream" together (me, naturally, off-key!). With Micah, Olivia and Emory, Mary and I rode in a horse-drawn carriage around the Club's grounds. All that was missing was snow! What a difference between Christmas 2013 when I was near death at Emory University Hospital and Christmas 2014 when, at the Dickens Dinner, I was exhilarated by my family, friends and life.

After Christmas, it took Mary and me over two weeks to take down 46 years of glorious Christmas decorations. An entire section of our storage room is dedicated to Christmas decorations, ornaments, elegant lights, collections, memorabilia, wreaths and unique family items accumulated lovingly over the years. Hopefully, our children and grandchildren will eventually enjoy these Christmas treasures. Christmas has always been very special in/to our family. Especially as my celebratory "first birthday" approached (i.e., one year after my heart transplant), Mary made Christmas 2014 for me one of the most loving and memorable ever!

On New Year's Eve, at exactly 7:17 pm (i.e., the moment a year earlier when I learned that I was "a go"), I called the CCU. On a speaker phone, I thanked my nurses again for their immense efforts in keeping me alive for those 70 extraordinary and challenging days in 2013. As I wished them all a Happy New Year, they extended their warmest regards for my "first birthday"! That day, I also thought profoundly about and prayed regularly for my generous and caring heart donor and his family. However, by then an extraordinary meeting with my donor's mother had been arranged. Quite wondrously, in a few days, that meeting would happen (Chapter XVI)!

CHAPTER XIV:
Year Two Challenges

"No matter how one's body is challenged, the human mind is our most fundamental and indefatigable resource"

—John F. Kennedy

My second year as a heart transplant recipient began with greater awareness of what to expect in terms of my body's proclivities and tendencies. I felt stronger and more confident that my body's danger zones had somewhat abated. With renewed optimism, my expectations for the year were more hale and hearty than they had been in some time. I envisioned some days where I would still feel unwell – but, at the same time, recognized that my coping skills were much better than in year one. Moreover, since some of my medications had been tapered, the harshest collateral effects on my body and mind seemed to have subsided. I felt buoyant in that I had survived the first year with neither rejection nor significant infections. All this portended a good "Year Two"!

In January and February 2015 it was unseasonably cold. Therefore, it became risky even to walk outside. Instead, with a surgical mask, I occasionally tried the treadmill at my Club where we live. However, given my compromised immune system, my doctors and I were always extremely alert to environments which might breed infections (i.e., workout facilities, indoor pools, movie theaters, airports/planes, cruises, etc.). Nevertheless, in late February/early March, I took a chance (once again, much to my doctors' chagrin!) – and, with Mary, took Alexander and Emory on a week-long Disney Cruise in the Caribbean. (A few years earlier, we had taken Micah and Olivia on a similar cruise.) Although it was only 14 months after my heart transplant, we had promised this trip to Alexander and Emory.

Whatever Disney does is magical. However, this long-awaited cruise with Alexander and Emory was *absolutely spectacular*. From time-to-time Mary and I struggled to keep-up with Alexander and Emory's non-stop activities and adventures on the magnificent *Disney Fantasy*. However, timely afternoon naps for us all helped Mary and me stay "afloat". Then, when we returned to Georgia, my entire family welcomed us with an emotional and heart-warming surprise party to celebrate my 70th birthday. My daughters, sons-in-law, grandchildren, brother, sister-in-law and cousins, Keith and Cathy, were all there. I had made it to my 70th birthday and, with my family, rejoiced that I was alive!

With spring in the air, I began to look forward to a re-birth of my golf game. It had been almost 3 years since I'd been able to swing my clubs comfortably and play a round of golf. Moreover, for the first time in over two years I had accepted an opportunity to lecture to college students. A trip to New York's Cornell University and Ithaca College had been arranged for mid-April. My spirits soared as I felt more athletic than I had in some time. On days when I felt especially well I pushed myself hard. I would exercise more, practice at the golf range and begin to swing a new tennis racquet which my daughter, Jennifer (an ALTA Champion), gave me for my 70th birthday. My reading became more focused and I began to devote significant time each day to prepare for my upcoming college lectures. Additionally, I began to revisit seriously the "list of 17" which I had scripted in CCU-409. Since I still dozed for an hour or two each afternoon, I began to feel strong enough to plan occasional evenings with friends. I even considered attending a college football game in the fall and, as such, purchased some (rather expensive!) tickets for the Notre Dame-Clemson game in October. For the first time in years, Mary and I went to a movie and our Club's St. Patrick's Day party where I raised a song or two to all my fine Irish friends. Despite Mary's chronic health problems and our concerns about our daughter's cancer risks, for the time-being I could actually see some "blue skies"! My grandchildren were thriving and my daughter, Heather, was in a new home in Old Greenwich, Connecticut. All told, it was wonderful to be busy and accomplishing some meaningful tasks again.

Then, suddenly, on March 25th, my fortunes changed; my health took a significant "hit". On that day, I was on the golf course and, in agony, had to discontinue playing. My symptoms included: my right foot burning as if it was on fire; numbness on my right side; distorted balance; and a throbbing headache. My golf friends helped me home and Mary, thinking I was having a stroke, promptly drove me to Emory University Hospital's ER.

Following a circuitous path, I was ultimately admitted to EUH. Eight days and countless doctors, multiple/insightful tests, pain medications, steroids and muscle relaxants later, my doctors determined that an area of my spine (between L3, L4 and L5 & S1) seemed to have contracted some type of infection causing "bulging and nerve roots"-type damage. Although I repeatedly insisted that the worst pain was in my right foot, ankle and large toe, my doctors discharged me with some meds. and a follow-up appointment with a pain doctor.

Over the next 5 weeks, I experienced *the worst pain of my life*! Notwithstanding all that I had been through over the past several years (and, in particular, the last 18 months), nothing could compare with the sheer agony of my right foot, ankle and large toe. The pain was extreme and my right foot, ankle and leg were swollen and discolored as if they had been burned. Any touch, even a gently-placed sheet at night, triggered untrammeled anguish. Without sleep, and although requiring transport in a wheelchair and golf cart, I still lectured and rose (albeit at times on one foot!) on schedule in mid-April at Cornell University and Ithaca College. For 2 ½ days, in severe pain, I taught Global Risk Management to some bright students on two magnificent college campuses.

Five weeks after my March hospitalization at EUH, and after seeing a pain doctor for spinal injections, there was still no relief from my foot and toe suffering. Finally, on April 27th when I was being readied in the Cath. Lab. for a

heart biopsy, I simply refused until a doctor had a serious
look at my excruciatingly painful right foot, ankle, leg and
toe. Remarkably, in about 5 seconds, one of my cardiac
docs. announced that I was suffering with gout! In fact,
gout was not an uncommon byproduct for heart transplant
patients and had simply been overlooked as the principal
cause of my "quandary" for over a month. Thankfully, I
was able to see a rheumatologist that day and begin appropriate medication to calm the pain in my right foot, ankle, leg and toe. However, I soon discovered that the gout
caused some broader nerve damage which, over the next
few months, was labeled Type II - Complex Regional Pain
Syndrome (CRPS).

Although by May some of my gout symptoms began to
retreat, my CRPS made it more difficult for me to walk.
My balance was also compromised and, taking new/much
stronger medications prescribed by my rheumatologist or
pain doctor, made me even less secure on my feet. Some
of the new meds. also disrupted my sleep and that, in turn,
made me more susceptible to unpleasant abdominal and
respiratory "viruses". Nevertheless, there was never a day
when, despite significant pain, I didn't give thanks for
my new miraculous gift and for the donor who gave me
life. I recognized that my pain, albeit reprehensible, reminded me that, as before, I would overcome this bump in

the road. Hence, I sought proactively broader remedies to my chronic foot and toe discomfort and balance dilemma. Finally, in early summer, I was introduced to an enlightened physical therapist at Emory Johns Creek Hospital. He, through intelligence, follow-up and polite persistence, began the arduous task of mitigating the destructive effects of my gout, related nerve damage and CRPS. I am deeply indebted to that talented, bright and compassionate physical therapist.

By mid-summer, I recognized that the sanguineness of spring would have to be postponed for a few months. I still could not play golf and, given balance issues and chronic foot and toe discomfort, I was reluctant to accept invitations to participate in various academic lectures, seminars and fora around the country. I did begin to write this book, but was often sidetracked by some renewed issues around Mary's health. In fact, given the frequency of my trips to EUH, I soon learned a new definition for mixed emotions. Namely, being ambivalent when greeted by name by doctors, nurses, technicians, staff, etc. as I roamed the halls of EUH!

In July, our daughters' families, Mary and I spent a week in the Historical Triangle known as Williamsburg, Jamestown and Yorktown, Virginia. Notwithstanding my inability to walk comfortably, each member of my family (including my 3 older grandchildren!), took turns escorting me by wheelchair through some wonderful colonial history. Here, too, despite my apprehensions each time I tried to stand, I was delighted simply to be on vacation with my family and cherishing our precious time together. Appendix G was photographed as we toured Williamsburg.

With physical therapy helping by summer's end, Mary and I decided in September to attend her 50th high school Reunion in St. Marys, Ohio. St. Marys is a small town in west-central Ohio. Mary was raised in that quaint midwestern town and, interestingly, it was where her father's family had settled when they arrived in the U.S. from Germany in 1849. Yet St. Marys was my wife's home town and, for that, I enjoyed seeing her joy and pride whenever we returned.

Unfortunately, for Mary's Reunion Weekend it rained heavily and was very cold. Still we both participated fully. It was most enjoyable to celebrate the Reunion's main event at the Club on Grand Lake St. Marys where Mary and I had had our wedding reception 46 years earlier. However, as the evening progressed, I began to feel quite ill – including a rising fever. Alarmed at the symptoms (i.e., given my exposed immune system, new heart, etc.),

Mary and I knew that we must seek top professional medical care as soon as possible. After saying our fond farewells to Mary's high school friends, we decided to drive 3 ½ hours to the Cleveland Clinic (CC). Our plans had been to travel east anyway to see some relatives – but, instead, we drove directly to the CC.*

After a two minute brief introduction in the ER, I was admitted immediately to the CC's heart transplant wing. Pneumonia was suspected and, if so, that presented for me a very serious risk. Mary and I were very disappointed that, after more than one and one half years, yet another problem had surfaced to disrupt my heart transplant recovery. At the CC, I was treated immediately by Iv with two alternating types of antibiotics to fight the suspected cause(s) of my pneumonia. Simultaneously, my blood was drawn regularly and, from same, samples taken and incubated to identify the type of infection(s). Thankfully, after 5 days in the CC, no virulent infections were discovered. Hence, with oral medications and instructions to followup as soon as possible with my doctors at EUH, I was discharged. Intriguingly, while at the CC, I was fortunate to be treated principally by one of the foremost authorities in the U.S. on heart failure. In due course, I hope that impressive M.D. will include my book in his library.

---

*   As noted earlier, The Cleveland Clinic is the premier cardiac hospital in the U.S.

By mid-October, I was able to conquer the pneumonia and, feeling better, began to consider a surprise visit to Connecticut for Halloween week. Recalling events in CCU-409 two years earlier (i.e., the night I thought I was having a fatal heart attack), I wanted to see my daughter/Heather's sons for Halloween. I booked a flight and surprised them for the Halloween week of events. Mary couldn't join me as she was preparing for abdominal surgery on the forthcoming Monday. Juxtaposing my three year-old grandson/William's costume as Batman, I dressed to battle the bad guys as Captain America! My 7 year-old grandson, Alexander, completed our "team" as a bold Ninja Warrior. Thankfully the weather was mild and our unique week together at Halloween parties, attending soccer games and trick-or-treating with my adorable grandsons was most memorable.

The day I returned from Connecticut, Mary and I were at EUH at 5:00 am. It was November 2nd and she was scheduled for abdominal surgery. The surgery went well except, shortly thereafter, a second abdominal operation was required. Unfortunately, that second surgery was followed by serious post op. neurological problems – including incredibly painful headaches and stroke-like symptoms. Therefore, in November and December, Mary spent nearly three weeks in a hospital room at EUH. Nevertheless, for Christmas, Mary and I flew to Heather's home in Old Greenwich, Connecticut. Simultaneously, Jennifer and her family had driven up from Roswell, GA. There, all together, we celebrated a wonderful Christmas. Naturally, on New Year's Eve (as with the prior year), I called the donor's mother and EUH's CCU. Then, on New Year's Day, with prayers and a birthday cake with two candles, my family and I observed my "second birthday".

Since my initial diagnosis (Chapter I), the phrase "looking forward to it" became an integral part of my daily vocabulary. In CCU-409, I actually built a list of the things which I expected to do once I returned home. In fact, by New Year's Day 2014 (i.e., the day I received the gift of life), there were 17 significant items on my list. Among those were this book, the Disney (and other) cruises, paying it forward (Chapter XV), honoring the donor (Chapter XVI), traveling to places Mary and I had yet to visit and, most importantly, enjoying my grandchildren in every aspect of their lives. In Year Two, even when sidetracked by some significant calamities, family, song, humor, positive conversations, faith and perseverance always seemed to make the days softer and the nights more tolerable. As I enter 2016, I recognize daily that I am an extraordinarily fortunate man. I have been blessed with a new strong and (each day I sense) very caring heart! After all, surrounded by my family and with my body mostly healed from the medical misfortunes of 2015, I'm looking forward to many more of my heart transplant "birthdays"! Perhaps, this spring, I may even be able to return to the golf course!

CHAPTER XV:
Paying It Forward

"You can't live a perfect day without doing something for someone who will never be able to repay you."

—John Wooden

Most of my adult life, I've believed in trying to perform as Mr. Wooden preached. Certainly, there have been times when I have succeeded and times where I have fallen short. Despite the monumental hurdles recorded in this book, I have striven to continue to embrace this magnanimous concept. In this Chapter, I will cover briefly how, where and for whom – since October 23, 2013 (the day I was admitted to EUH's CCU) — I have tried/am trying to "pay it forward".

Since October 23, 2013, the most important contribution that I've made has been to stay alive for my family. That's not intended to be self-righteous; rather, it's based on my deep love for my family. Yes, indeed, they are all strong and can survive without me. However, the adults in my immediate family told me "we want you around". Simultaneously, my grandchildren would add "G-Dad – you're awesome, we need you to be with us". Per se that's not paying it forward; yet, at many times it gave me a sense that, through them – if I stayed strong – I would be paying it forward.

The next most important item is this book. <u>Resolute: My Quest For A New Heart,</u> embodies many of the attributes necessary to stay alive under extreme, life-threatening circumstances. However, without an organ donor, I would not have survived! Woven throughout this book are numerous expressions of my gratitude for the young man who had the courage and consideration to become an organ donor. That selfless act was the most humane and magnanimous thing to which any individual may commit. Therefore, my sincerest hope is that my book will help generate many more organ donors so that other patients' impossible dreams may also be fulfilled.

After I had been in the CCU for about 1 1/2 months, the CCU's Director of Nursing, asked me if I would accept being interviewed by a senior executive from the American Nurses Credentialing Center (ANCC). EUH was being considered for "Magnet" status. After the Director explained the importance of being a Magnet hospital, I told her that "of course I would accept the interview".

A Magnet-designated hospital is one in which its nurses have been recognized by the ANCC after demonstrating excellence in patient care in over 35 areas throughout the hospital. It is a very prestigious appointment which carries with it substantial benefits to patients, nurses, doctors and the community at large. Only 6% of hospitals in the U.S. are considered Magnet qualified.

I understood that only a small number of patients in each part of the hospital were selected to be interviewed. Despite being ungroomed (no shower, shave or haircut for over 6 weeks) and, of course, being attired inelegantly in a plain hospital gown, I rose to the occasion (not literally, of course!). Without hesitation and quite persuasively I applauded my nurses, demonstrated specific areas where they had excelled, recreated instances of extraordinary kindness and, of course, fully supported their eligibility for Magnet status. On the day I left Mason House for home, banners flew everywhere in and around EUH. As Mary and I passed some of those banners as she drove me home from Mason House, I pumped my fist in the air and cheered heartily. My well-deserved nurses had become "Magnets" and, at least tangentially in a small way, I'd paid it forward for both them and their future patients.

Each year the <u>Atlanta Journal - Constitution</u> (AJC), Atlanta's largest newspaper, presents an award to Atlanta's finest nurse. The paper's audience recommends and the AJC's editors decide. As I was leaving The Floor, one of my favorite nurses, asked me to consider recommending the CCU's Director of Nursing. Instead, I recommended ALL the CCU nurses. When my letter was received, the AJC told me that, for 2014, it was a "done deal". In fact, from the moment my letter was received, my CCU nurses had won! Indeed, as I mentioned in my letter "over the 70 days of my intensive care in the CCU, I had received the finest care by skilled, devoted and competent nurses".

By mid-June, as I regained some strength, Mary and I felt compelled to host a "tribute dinner" at our club for CCU's finest. Fifteen nurses were invited; fourteen attended. (The nurse who couldn't join us was in India vacationing with her family.) Mary took charge of many of the event's details – including: elegant invitations; a specially dedicated/beautiful room for dinner; appetizing hors d'oeuvres; and the best table cloths, silver and plates that the club could offer. For music, my son-in-law, Heith, burned a CD with some of my favorite and CCU - memorable songs. The cocktail hour and dinner were grand and, deeply, Mary and I paid tribute to these special people (13 women and one man). When I commented that "the dew of compassion is often revealed best in a nurse's tears" (from Lord Byron), some (including our wait staff) wiped away a few tears. When the evening finally ended, the nurses told Mary and me that "something like this had never been done before". In turn, Mary and I expressed to them "our extreme gratitude, profound respect and deepest affection".

At this point, I'll return to "The Red Phone". My readers should recall that it was mentioned earlier. After going home, and following my nurses' Tribute Dinner, Mary and I decided to find an appropriate painting for the cardiac wing of EUH. To quote William James: "The greatest use of life is to spend it for something that outlasts it". Therefore, on October 30th, 2014 (my daughter Jennifer's 41st birthday) we presented our painting. It was simply entitled "The Red Phone". Those in attendance were EUH's CEO and a group of doctors and nurses from EUH's CCU. One of the last sentences of my remarks that day is worth repeating.

When your challenges seem insurmountable and you need *Him* most, we hope that *His* red phone will ring promptly and resoundingly for you.

Today, that painting hangs in EUH's Cardiac Cath. Lab. I know that it will "outlast" me. Most importantly, I hope that it will bring hope to those waiting for the gift of life.

Before year-end 2014, Mary and I made a gift to Emory's Nell Hodgson Woodruff School of Nursing. We did so to help develop future nurses. Hopefully, when educated, trained and seasoned properly, some will eventually work in the CCU. Sanguinely, they may hear about a man who, until he was too weak, sang each day to their predecessors.

Another "pay it forward" that I should mention is mentoring. The latter has been my life's passion since my graduate school days at Notre Dame. I have always enjoyed helping others to succeed. That passion was evidenced throughout my personal and professional lives. Some whom I've mentored have become senior luminaries in the private, public and academic sectors. Even when I was in CCU-409 waiting to live, I encouraged young doctors to stop-by for "coffee hour" with this sedulous and well-traveled man. Today, at a few colleges and universities, I still enjoy helping students grasp some of the world's nuances and fulfill their dreams.

<u>At least for now</u>, my final pay-it-forward involves my donor's family. That <u>very</u> <u>significant</u> topic deserves a Chapter of its own. Hence, Chapter XVI.

In closing, it's worth mentioning that during my long-wait in CCU-409 I focused each day on how/where to pay-it-forward. It became a mental exercise which I treasured. Save sharing a few of my ideas with my wife and a handful of nurses, I savored those "imaginations" as exclusively mine. Some reflections were part of the "list of 17" mentioned in my previous Chapter. I drew strength by promising God and others that, as long as my heart beats, I will always try to pay it forward!

CHAPTER XVI:

Honoring The Donor

"Remember me for the life I lived and for the life I gave"

—*My Heart Donor*

The quote above appears at the foot of my heart donor's grave! Mary and I have been to his grave nestled in a small town in Georgia. We prayed there and left beautiful flowers at the grave site. On the day we visited (May 4, 2015), we also visited my donor's family and his high school. At his high school, we met with his former advisers and teachers and, of course, current students.* We also visited the grocery store where he worked and, soon, was to become an Assistant Manager. While there, we conversed with his former boss, colleagues and

---

* Wondrously, within days of my visit, I learned that many of the high school students with whom I met became organ donors.

friends. <u>All</u> with whom we met loved the young man, described him as fun-loving, bright, thoughtful and, kindly and affectionately, called him "boss". It was clear to Mary and me that my heart donor had a special joy for life and had been a wonderful son, student, friend and colleague.

Essentially my donor's life and mine "connected" on December 30, 2013. That night my heart donor perished in a horrible accident. Thankfully for me (and hundreds of other recipients of his organs, tissues, bones, ligaments, tendons, etc.), the EMS team was at the accident site very quickly. Of course, I had no idea of all this until late the next day when I learned that there was a "match" for me. Since some of my previous Chapters cover in detail the course of events since that miraculous news on December 31, 2013, I will fast forward to the orchestration of/initial meeting with my heart donor's mother and step father. Remarkably, that meeting took place one year <u>to the day</u> after they buried their precious son.

On Valentine's Day 2014, six weeks after my heart transplant, I began trying to correspond with my heart donor's family. I was so very grateful that I wanted to reach out and thank them for their son's amazing generosity. My letter was cleared through multiple "channels" (e.g., EUH's Chaplain, Donate Life GA., etc.) – and, six weeks later, finally delivered to my heart donor's mother. When we finally met on January 3, 2015, she shared with me that my letter "had given her hope to go on living." As we embraced on that rainy and cold January day at Donate Life Georgia's offices, tears streamed down our faces. Only then, for real, could I actually taste her inconceivable loss! Here was a woman who was my younger daughter's age (late thirties) and who had given birth to her oldest son in her late teens. Twenty years later, that boy had died horrifically. After our meeting, Mary and I invited my heart donor's mother and step father to lunch. Over lunch, that loving lady constantly held my wrist; she simply wanted to feel her son's pulse!

After our January meeting, my heart donor's mother and I continued to correspond regularly by phone calls, e-mails and texts. I learned that my heart donor was: his mother's "best friend"; the oldest of 8 children; fond of music (especially playing the guitar); very close to his family and enjoyed shepherding his younger siblings; a hard worker; and "a very good kid." I also learned that the one thing that has given his mother comfort was "knowing that others lived through her son's selflessness." Quite generously, on February 7, 2015, my heart donor's mother wrote to Mary as follows:

Please know that I thank you! I thank you for being the wife, nurse and caregiver you were for Lance. And I thank you for now loving a piece of my son. I can see the love you have for Lance and that makes me happy to know a piece of my son is surrounded by love.

In May, encouraged by my heart donor's mother (and as noted earlier in this Chapter), Mary and I traveled to my heart donor's small Georgia town. That day (May 4, 2015), in addition to what I referred earlier, I also consoled my heart donor's grandmother. Most of that day she would cradle her ear against my chest and insist on listening to her grandson's heart. Each time, as she wept softly, that loving grandmother kept apologizing for getting makeup on my shirt! How fragile she was; how tender those moments!

Before leaving that Georgia town, I gave my heart donor's mother an EKG. It was mine but, of course, had also been her son's. The mother had a copy of her son's EKG taken just before his heart was removed. That EKG was placed on a wall in her son's room. My identical EKG now hangs and "lives" in that room next to her son's!

The following e-mail (dated January 4, 2015 to my heart donor's mother) summarizes cogently my enormous appreciation of/gratitude for my January 1, 2014 miracle:

> Through me your son will see my 5 grandchildren grow and prosper. Through me, each will know of your son; each will appreciate who he was and what he's done for their G-Dad.

Honoring the heart donor was included at the top of my CCU "list of 17". After my heart transplant, it became even more important for me to meet the donor's family. When we met, I gained strength from my heart donor's mother. More importantly, through her relief in meeting my wife and me, some of her grief seemed to melt away. She felt that somehow, in me, her son was living on. She sensed that I would cherish her son's heart and use it in a fruitful and compassionate way. To her, that was vitally important in coping with her anguish and, despite her tremendous loss, finding ways to move forward. In a letter to Mary and me at Christmas 2015, my heart donor's mother wrote:

> For everything there is a reason and I truly believe the reason for our journey was because your family needed two grandparents to continue making memories of a lifetime with some very lucky, special and blessed children and grandchildren.

Going forward, I hope that UNOS will find ways to encourage attentively receptive interactions between donors and recipients. I wish that Donate Life Georgia and other similar organizations would be more proactive in facilitating appropriate correspondence between donors and recipients. There is no reason, for instance, why letters between donors and recipients take so many weeks to process through various so-called "privacy channels". Sometimes those letters (as with mine) offer timely support to devastated parents, relatives, etc. and, by so doing, allow them merely to cope with yet another day of grief.

For the rest of our lives, Mary and I will stay in-touch with my donor's mother and her family. My family and close friends will learn of the young man who gave his heart to me so that I could live.

Epilogue

As I've written this book, I've felt inspired and invigorated. Inspired by some unique insights (perhaps from above!) which kept me up at night; invigorated by finally getting "this" off my chest. By "this" I don't mean the burden of not telling my story; rather, it's the relief one feels when a promise has been fulfilled. After all, I had promised God and my immediate family that I would write deeply from my new heart about this remarkable quest. *I have, indeed*!

I've taken a unique ride – one which very few have experienced. Indeed, heart transplants are still quite rare. When I ask other heart transplant recipients what it's been like for them, the answer is always "only those who have made this trip will ever know". A road such as this will lead you into a world which, in all respects, is unearthly, tormenting and, yet, strangely satisfying. The struggle will challenge you to your physical, emotional, psychological and spiritual limits. At times, death was always looming!

Now to the positives of this incredible experience. Along this journey, I have learned more about my family, friends and myself. I have gained a new appreciation for the value of time and understood better my priorities. I recognize – and am most grateful for – the extraordinary opportunity for a second chance. Although I cannot comprehend why a mature, happy, hard-working and kind 20 year-old man died to give me life, I have rationalized that, for some reason, God decided that I should have more time. In turn, I have promised Him a quid pro quo!

From the bottom of my heart, I hope that my readers will (if not already) become organ donors. I wish that they will also encourage others along this most noble of paths. I also trust that those readers waiting for a heart transplant will benefit from the messages in my book. Specifically, faith, family, resoluteness, courage, humor, song and a lust for many more tomorrows. As you listen for "The Red Phone" to chime for you, always keep your mind, soul and heart open to miracles.

APPENDIX A:

Micah's Essay

My Greatest Person
By Micah Rodman

My Granddad believed that he could "reach a star, an unreachable star," in his life. He knew that if he had strength, knowledge, and enough faith, that he could reach the impossible dream of new life. My Granddad ("G-Dad") survived almost three long months in a hospital waiting for a heart transplant. Despite the long wait, my G-Dad's attitude and spirit stayed strong as an ox, and never stopped believing that a new heart would come, giving him a new life. Besides his courage, he never lost his faith, nor his desire for knowledge while in the hospital. My GDad's favorite song to play while in the hospital, and the song that best suits him is called "The Impossible Dream" — "*That one man scorned, and covered with his scars, still strove with his last ounce of courage.*" Doctors, nurses, and patients around him, could hear the strong but soothing sound of his voice singing that song.

During my G-Dad's stay in the hospital for three months, "*to beat the unbeatable foe*", he would never pout about his pain, or cry about his suffering. My G-Dad showed strength through every test and procedure he endured, including the actual transplant. When I visited him, I would always sit next to him in bed, holding onto his cold, soft hands to see if he was still shaking or if he was getting stronger; even on his rough days, he showed me only strength and determination. One day I want have that kind of strength, able take on any challenge, any "*unbeatable foe*". Additionally, once my G-Dad was given the gift of his new heart, he remained strong and determined push through the pain of many months of strenuous rehabilitation and awful anti-rejection medications. Moreover, even now when he comes to our house, he parks at the bottom of our long hill a walks up, trying to push his body and get his full strength back.

In addition to strength, my G-Dad has demonstrated faith in God in many ways. Every time I entered the hospital room, I saw him in a little, bleak, boring hospital room, with no windows to the outside world. The room always smelled and tasted stale and like death. He was always lying in bed with tubes and wires coming in and out of his chest and arms. Despite the depressing nature of his environment, every time I visited him, G-Dad greeted me with a huge smile, and told me to keep on believing. "*No matter how far, to fight for the right and without question or pause.*" Also, to keep up his spirits and to show his doctors and nurses that he still had hope, he would sing to the nurses and say that he would be home for Christmas. For example, one song that he would always sing to his Irish nurse was the Notre Dame Fight Song. He would sing so loud and proud, that the patients in the other rooms would hear and chuckle. Even after the third month in the hospital, never leaving his bed, he maintained his belief that God would deliver. He truly believed that God would deliver a new heart before Christmas, and so he used to sing "I'll Be Home For Christmas" at the top of his spirited lungs. When the rest of us began to lose hope, my G-Dad told us to hold onto our undoubting faith.

Beyond his strength of heart and faith, my G-Dad also has strength of mind. He firmly believes that the most important distance in life is between your ears. Even in a hospital room, he never stopped reading or working on the computer to keep up with his knowledge. My G-Dad has always had a thirst for knowledge, and the betterment of his life . He was the first member of his family to attend a four-year college. After graduating from college, he was offered a full scholarship the University of Notre Dame to receive his Master's degree. After receiving his Master's Notre Dame, he traveled the world with an international job, picking up new languages and learning about new cultures. During my G-Dad's stay in the hospital, I chose to do my Fifth grade Heritage Project on him and his Portuguese heritage. Every day, he provided me new information about his heritage and the country of Portugal. His knowledge was never-ending and very detailed, and he would email me every night (and I mean night!!). My G-Dad is the most learned and knowledgeable person in my world.

In conclusion, my G-Dad is courageous, faithful, and very knowledgeable. He is my wisdom, my strength, and my faith. He is my greatest and he reached "The Impossible Dream" of getting a new heart at almost 69 years old! *"Yes, and he'll reach the unreachable star."* I hope you enjoyed hearing about my incredible G-Dad, the greatest person in my world.

APPENDIX B:

Christmas Day 2013
With My Family

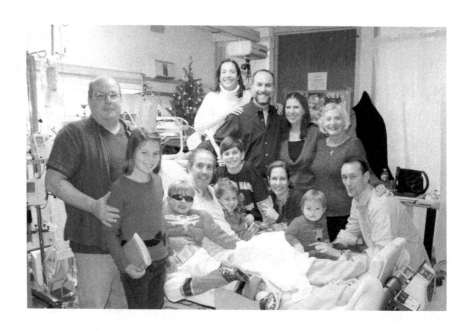

Back row: Heather, Heith, Melissa, Mary
Front Row: Scott, Olivia, Alexander, me, Emory,
Micah, Jennifer, William, Christopher.
Appendix B depicts my family and me on Christmas Day 2013.

APPENDIX C:
First Waking In The ICU With Mary

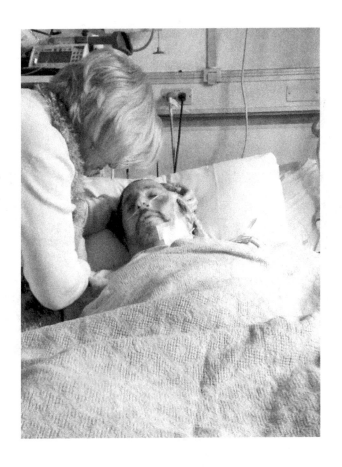

APPENDIX D:

*My Daughters
With Me In The ICU*

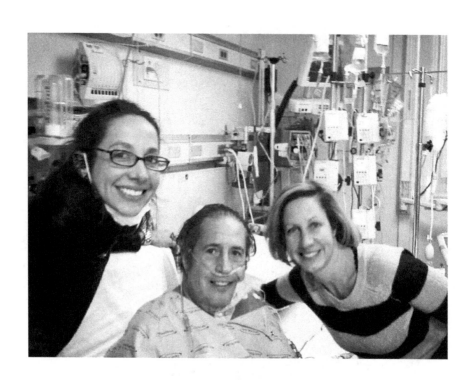

APPENDIX E:

Arriving Home

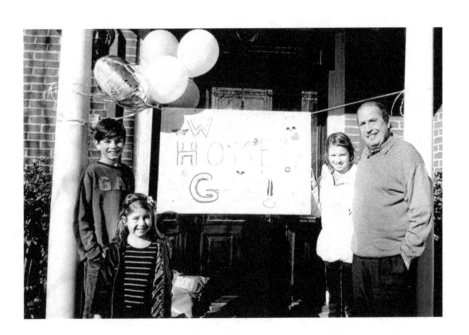

APPENDIX F:

Thanksgiving 2014

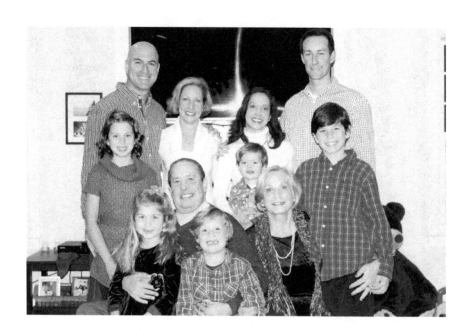

APPENDIX G:

July 2015 In Williamsburg, VA

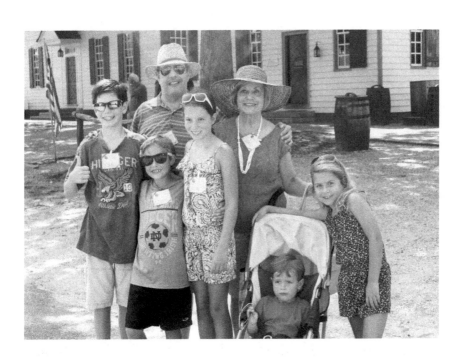

Acknowledgements
"In perpetuum gratias"

Notwithstanding my mental and spiritual commitments to write this book, there were times when I doubted my ability to stay the course. At those times, I was encouraged most by my wife, Mary. However, there were also two others – both close friends – who, perhaps unbeknownst to them, made me feel that this book was important. Gary Balsam and Chuck Schneider encouraged me to tell my story. To them, I am most grateful.

In terms of medical advice, I want to thank an exceptional R.N. and P.A. Both in the hospital as I waited for a heart, as well as from time-to-time as I wrote this book, Cheryl Lee and Gabriel Najarro, respectively, helped me understand better my condition, procedures and treatment. I will always make room for them in my new heart.

Others I should acknowledge as a group are the kind and thoughtful members of St. Brigid Catholic Church and its benevolent Prayer Quilt Ministry. Also, during this long ordeal so many friends and acquaintances in Country Club of The South were exceptionally kind and generous to Mary and me. From the bottom of my heart – I thank you all!

On a broader scale, knowing that relatives, friends and former colleagues from around the world were praying for Mary and me made us feel as if there was always a candle glowing for us somewhere. That iridescence, as well as the entreaties which I honestly sensed, ignited a flame which gave me strength to carry on. Gradually, the light from that flame also drew me back to my childhood Catholic roots. For those prayers, as well as my spiritual "return", I will always be *in perpetuum gratias*!

CPSIA information can be obtained
at www.ICGtesting.com
Printed in the USA
LVHW081342210319
611413LV00036B/693/P